T0322987

UNDERSTANDING
MENTAL HEALTH CARE

UNDERSTANDING MENTAL HEALTH CARE

CRITICAL ISSUES IN PRACTICE

MARC ROBERTS

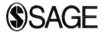

Los Angeles | London | New Delhi
Singapore | Washington DC | Melbourne

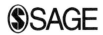

Los Angeles | London | New Delhi
Singapore | Washington DC | Melbourne

SAGE Publications Ltd
1 Oliver's Yard
55 City Road
London EC1Y 1SP

SAGE Publications Inc.
2455 Teller Road
Thousand Oaks, California 91320

SAGE Publications India Pvt Ltd
B 1/I 1 Mohan Cooperative Industrial Area
Mathura Road
New Delhi 110 044

SAGE Publications Asia-Pacific Pte Ltd
3 Church Street
#10-04 Samsung Hub
Singapore 049483

Editor: Alex Clabburn
Editorial assistant: Jade Grogan
Production editor: Katie Forsythe
Copyeditor: Rosemary Campbell
Proofreader: William Baginsky
Indexer: Silvia Benvenuto
Marketing manager: Tamara Navaratnam
Cover design: Wendy Scott
Typeset by: C&M Digitals (P) Ltd, Chennai, India
Printed in the UK

Library of Congress Control Number: 2017957932

British Library Cataloguing in Publication data

A catalogue record for this book is available from the British Library

ISBN 978-1-5264-0447-3
ISBN 978-1-5264-0448-0 (pbk)

CONTENTS

ABOUT THE AUTHOR

Dr Marc Roberts is a researcher, writer and lecturer with extensive and varied experience working in mental health practice and education. In addition to having clinical experience in mental health care he also has an academic background in philosophy. His research is therefore concerned with the way in which critical thinking, critical reflection and philosophy more generally can contribute to the theory and practice of contemporary mental health care.

ACKNOWLEDGEMENTS

I would like to thank Becky Taylor, Charlène Burin and the rest of the team at SAGE for their work in commissioning this book and their support throughout its development. In addition, I wish to thank the staff at Lichfield public library for providing me with an environment in which to work. Finally, I would once again like to thank Ruth, John and Philippa for their ongoing encouragement throughout the writing process, and without whom this book would not have been possible.

INTRODUCTION

Contemporary mental health care is a complex and contested field of professional practice. What were once considered acceptable and productive ways of understanding and responding to mental distress are increasingly subject to critical examination. Such critical work is not only being conducted by the variety of professionals who practise within mental health services, but it is also being carried out by people who use those services. As a consequence, the authority of mental health professionals and the legitimacy of their interventions are the focus of ongoing critical consideration, and those who experience mental distress are increasingly calling for greater involvement in how their experiences are understood and addressed. Moreover, in response to the requirement to practise in an evidence-based, collaborative and recovery-focused way with those who use mental health services, practitioners are required as never before to appraise and justify the theory, research and evidence which informs the whole range of their work.

To provide informed, effective and responsive mental health care in this challenging and changing context, it is therefore necessary for mental health professionals to develop an understanding of, and engage actively with, the critical issues which characterise that context. Such engagement not only enables practitioners to consider critically the breadth of information which informs their work, but it is also necessary for the development of a critical awareness of how their own assumptions, values and beliefs may affect their practice in both productive and non-productive ways. Indeed, an engagement with critical issues in mental health care is essential for preventing potentially ineffective, dogmatic and paternalistic mental health care by questioning, challenging and seeking to change that which does not withstand critical examination, especially in response to contemporary research and evidence, the emergence of new theoretical perspectives and the innovative work of those who use mental health services.

The aim of this book is therefore to introduce, and facilitate an active engagement with, the critical issues that characterise contemporary mental health care. It is written primarily for mental health professionals and those who, in the course of their work, encounter people who experience mental distress. In addition, it will be of use to students undertaking a professional mental health qualification (or those pursuing a course of study that has a mental health care component) and for professionals who are returning to practice. Moreover, the practice-based character of the book, and the numerous case studies and activities used throughout, means that it can be employed as a resource by lecturers and clinical mentors involved in mental health education. Finally, in so far as many of the critical issues examined are informed by the work of the service user/survivor movement, this book may also be of interest to those people who experience mental distress.

The purpose of Chapter 1, 'Critical Issues in Mental Health Care', is to examine the significance of critical issues in mental health care. In the context of the tendency for certain approaches to mental distress to become dominant, it will consider how an active engagement with those issues is central to becoming an informed, self-aware and proactive practitioner who is responsive to the needs of people who use mental health services. In addition, it will reflect upon the manner in which this engagement requires the development of a variety of intellectual skills including an ability to consider critical questions, to engage in analysis and to use the capacity to reason. Moreover, while an engagement with critical issues is commonly thought of as being a purely intellectual activity, this chapter will suggest that it also requires the possession of a number of emotional qualities such as an openness of mind, an emotional self-awareness and the possession of courage.

Chapter 2, 'Causes of Mental Distress', is concerned with what contributes to the emergence and maintenance of mental distress and how such distress is understood more generally. It will begin by examining what has variously been referred to as the biological, medical or biomedical model of mental distress, which has been, and continues to be, vigorously debated and disputed. This chapter will then consider the emerging psychological and, in particular, trauma-informed approach to mental distress in which such distress is understood as a meaningful response to a range of traumatic and adverse events that can occur at various stages of an individual's life. Finally, this chapter will examine how a multiplicity of social, economic and political factors can profoundly influence and determine the social and material conditions of people's lives and, in doing so, contribute to the emergence and maintenance of mental distress throughout the course of those lives.

The aim of Chapter 3, 'Psychiatric Diagnosis', is to reflect upon a variety of critical issues surrounding psychiatric diagnosis. It will begin by considering the legitimacy of existing diagnostic categories and the extent to which they accurately identify, and draw clear boundaries between, supposedly distinct biologically based 'mental disorders'. Set against the notion that psychiatric diagnosis is a value-free enterprise, this chapter will then examine the manner in which a variety of social, cultural and historical values and norms are implicated in the diagnostic categories used in mental health care. Moreover, it will conclude by considering an alternative to psychiatric diagnosis that is referred to as psychological formulation or simply formulation. In doing so, this chapter will examine the way in which the thoughts, feelings and behaviours that are associated with mental distress may be understood as meaningful once they are situated in the unique context of a person's life history and current circumstances.

Chapter 4, 'Psychiatric Drugs', is concerned with a variety of critical issues surrounding the use of psychiatric drugs and the manner in which they are thought to work. It will begin by examining the widespread belief that psychiatric drugs work by targeting and correcting the biological dysfunctions or chemical imbalances that supposedly underlie the emergence and maintenance of mental distress. However, in contrast to the understanding of psychiatric drugs as precise medications or 'magic bullets' that target and correct chemical imbalances, this chapter will then discuss the notion that they are powerful psychoactive substances which produce a range of altered states and non-specific physiological and psychological effects. In doing so, it will consider the implications of these two ways of thinking about psychiatric drugs for how they are used in mental health care and for the character of the clinical and therapeutic relationship between practitioners and people who are prescribed psychiatric drugs.

The purpose of Chapter 5, 'Psychological Therapies', is to examine a variety of critical issues surrounding the use of psychological therapies. It will begin by considering the effectiveness of those interventions and the way in which the quality of the relationship that is established with people experiencing mental distress can influence this effectiveness. Moreover, despite the diverse range of available psychological therapies, many of them are said to possess an individualistic orientation in so far as they seek to facilitate change within the individual. This chapter will therefore move on to discuss the social and political implications of this individualistic orientation, as well as its potential limitations, for a productive understanding and response to mental distress. In contrast to the individualistic focus of various psychological therapies, this chapter will conclude by examining a variety of emerging initiatives that can be understood as being consistent with the field of practice that is known as community psychology.

Chapter 6, 'Service User/Survivor Involvement', is concerned with a variety of critical issues surrounding the involvement of mental health service users/survivors in the provision of those services. It will begin by reflecting upon the experiences of people who have used mental health services and the range of concerns that they have about the mental health system. In so far as the concerns of those who use mental health services have been influential in the formation of a service user/ survivor movement, this chapter will then examine the varied objectives and activities of that movement. Moreover, while the requirement to involve service users/ survivors in all aspects of mental health care is regarded as a significant achievement, this chapter will conclude by considering the extent to which it can be understood as meaningful, rather than being tokenistic, and the variety of barriers that may obstruct the inclusive, collaborative and transformative involvement of service users/survivors in the mental health system.

The aim of Chapter 7, 'Recovery', is to consider a variety of critical issues surrounding recovery in contemporary mental health care. While recovery has been understood in a variety of ways, this chapter will begin by reflecting upon how it is often formulated by those with personal experience of that process. It will then examine the manner in which recovery, through being adopted by the mental health system, is said to have been co-opted by and assimilated into that system. In doing so, this chapter will consider how the recovery-focused reorientation of mental health services has entailed, among other things, the marginalisation of the way in which recovery is formulated by those with experience of that process. Finally, despite the suggested co-option of recovery, this chapter will conclude by examining how personal accounts of recovery can enable mental health professionals to consider the conditions which are conducive to recovery and what they can do in their practice to establish such conditions.

1

CRITICAL ISSUES IN
MENTAL HEALTH CARE

CHAPTER AIMS

By the end of this chapter you will be able to:

- assess the importance of engaging with critical issues in mental health care;
- distinguish the intellectual skills associated with an engagement with critical issues in mental health care;
- distinguish the emotional qualities associated with an engagement with critical issues in mental health care.

INTRODUCTION

👥 CASE STUDY

Nadia has recently returned to work as a mental health professional after a number of years and has been surprised by the variety of questions, debates and disputes that now characterise mental health care. Of course, she is aware that there have always been critical concerns about psychiatry but these were largely treated as historical disputes that characterised the 1960s and which were commonly presented as having been resolved by developments in biological and pharmacological approaches to mental distress. However, she is now discovering that the theory and practice of contemporary mental health care is subject to sustained critique from a variety of sources. In particular, Nadia has noticed that critical concerns about existing approaches to mental distress are not only being conducted by those who work within mental health services, but they are also being systematically raised by people who use those services. While she feels that such developments may add a degree of complexity to her professional practice, she is excited by the opportunities that they bring to question, challenge and potentially change mental health care in more productive and responsive ways.

As Nadia in the above case study has recently discovered, contemporary mental health care is an increasingly contested and dynamic field of professional practice. What were once considered acceptable and productive ways of understanding and responding to mental distress are being challenged, both by those who work within and those who use mental health services. The authority of mental health professionals, the legitimacy of their knowledge base and the effectiveness of their interventions are subject to ongoing critical examination, and those who use mental health services are increasingly calling for greater involvement in how their experiences are understood and addressed. Indeed, the basic presuppositions and the clinical interventions that characterise contemporary mental health practice are subject to question in a way not seen in any other area of health care. Of course, there are concerns and debates in other areas but these rarely concern the theoretical foundations, therapeutic practices or very existence of the field of practice under consideration. For example, while various issues of concern may be raised in other branches of medicine (such as the length of waiting lists, the quality of practitioners' training and the adequacy of available resources and equipment), few would oppose the general purpose or existence of those medical specialities. As Bracken and Thomas (2001) suggest, it is difficult to imagine an anti-paediatrics, post-cardiology or critical neurology movement. However, the existence of the so-called **anti-psychiatry movement** and, more recently, the **critical psychiatry movement** illustrates how a sustained engagement with a variety of critical concerns has been, and continues to be, a feature of psychiatry and mental health care.

The purpose of this chapter is therefore to introduce you to the significance of critical issues in mental health care for your professional practice. It will begin by considering how an awareness of, and active engagement with, those issues is fundamental to becoming an informed, self-aware and proactive mental health professional who is responsive to the needs of those who use mental health services. In particular, this chapter will suggest that the importance of such engagement can be understood in the context of the tendency for certain approaches to mental distress to become dominant and to be viewed as self-evident, unquestionable and even natural. We shall then consider how an engagement with the principles and practices that characterise mental health care requires the development of a variety of cognitive capabilities or intellectual skills. While various intellectual skills have been proposed, this chapter will examine three that are of particular significance: an ability to consider critical questions, to engage in analysis and to use the capacity to reason. While an engagement with critical issues in any area of human inquiry is commonly thought of as being a purely intellectual activity, this chapter will suggest that it also requires the possession of a number of affective capabilities or emotional qualities. While a variety of emotional qualities have been proposed, we shall examine three that can be understood as being of particular significance for an engagement with critical issues in mental health care: an intellectual receptivity or openness of mind, an emotional self-awareness and, finally, the possession of courage.

WHY CRITICAL ISSUES IN MENTAL HEALTH CARE?

﷼ CASE STUDY

Since qualifying as a mental health professional a little under two years ago, Sophie has become increasingly interested in the debates that characterise contemporary mental health care. At lunchtime earlier today she was discussing her recent reading around some of these critical issues with her colleague Callum and the significance that they may have for their mental health practice. While Callum acknowledged that these issues sounded interesting, he was unsure of their relevance for the clinical area. Contemporary mental health care, he maintained, is an increasingly complex, challenging and pressurised area in which the role of practitioners is to respond to the needs of those who use mental health services in a safe, effective and efficient manner. While an engagement with critical issues in mental health care may have some value in an academic context, he suggested that it has minimal relevance for their everyday practice. Rather than spending time reflecting on practice and thinking about critical issues, Callum concluded by proposing that they should simply be focused on 'getting things done'.

Although contemporary mental health care is characterised by a variety of critical issues, the importance of developing an awareness of these issues may not be immediately clear. In the context of challenging and pressurised mental health settings it is not uncommon to develop a sense that mental health care, as suggested by Callum in the above case study, should be exclusively concerned with 'getting things done'. Indeed, it has been suggested that in so far as modern health care environments are increasingly task-orientated, and characterised by an ongoing drive to maximise efficiency in order to meet a range of health care targets, a culture can arise in which the importance of 'thinking', and of critical thinking and reflection in particular, can be marginalised at the expense of 'doing' (Thompson & Thompson 2008; Roberts & Ion 2015). Influenced by a health care culture that is focused on getting things done, and continually seeking to do so in the most efficient manner possible, an engagement with critical issues in mental health care can therefore come to be seen as a distraction, annoyance or unaffordable luxury at best. Moreover, in so far as it requires a reconsideration of existing ways of thinking and doing things, it has also been suggested that such critically reflective activity can come to be seen as an unproductive, undesirable and even unacceptable challenge to the aims, objectives and efficient functioning of the organisations in which health care is provided (Schön 1983).

In contrast to such concerns and characterisations, an engagement with critical issues in mental health care can be understood as being fundamental to becoming a practitioner who is responsive to the needs of those who use mental health services. To begin to understand how, it is productive to recognise that a variety of frameworks, models and **paradigms** have been used to comprehend mental distress and other societies, cultures and historical periods have understood and responded to such experiences in different and sometimes radically divergent ways (Foucault 2001; Scull 2016). Despite this diversity, there is an enduring tendency for certain approaches to mental distress to become favoured by individual practitioners, by the professional bodies and organisations with which they are associated and by the cultural and historical periods to which those individuals, professional bodies and organisations belong. However, the reasons why any one particular approach to mental distress becomes dominant is complex and contested. Such a dominance cannot, for example, simply be attributed to a supposed theoretical and therapeutic superiority over other ways of understanding and responding to mental distress. Rather, it has been argued that in any sphere of human inquiry a range of social, political and historical factors contribute to the establishment, maintenance and dominance of certain ways of understanding and responding to human experience while simultaneously marginalising, delegitimising and excluding alternative ways of understanding and responding to that experience (Foucault 1981).

CONCEPT SUMMARY: THE TECHNOLOGICAL MODEL OF MENTAL DISTRESS

It has been suggested that a particular approach to mental distress has come to dominate contemporary mental health care and, while it is the focus of critical consideration in some areas, is often uncritically maintained by many as being self-evident (Boyle 2011; Bracken *et al.* 2012). This dominant approach, or what has been referred to as the technological model of mental distress, is largely individualistic in so far as it understands that distress as primarily having its origin 'within' the individual, as a manifestation of some form of underlying biological dysfunction or psychological deficit. In doing so, it proposes that the most appropriate way to respond to that distress is through the expert application of various forms of technical intervention such as psychiatric medication or cognitive behavioural therapy.

It has been argued, however, that understanding and responding to mental distress by adopting this approach can have a variety of negative effects for those who use mental health services. By conceptualising mental distress as primarily having its origin within the individual, the technological model can obscure and even neglect how a variety of social and economic factors can contribute to the emergence and maintenance of that distress. Moreover, by prioritising professional understandings and responses to mental distress, the technological model not only minimises the personal meaning that such distress may have for a person, but it can also marginalise the expertise that the person may have obtained as a result of seeking to understand and respond to their particular experience of mental distress (Coles *et al.* 2015).

While the tendency for any one particular approach to mental distress to become dominant can have a range of negative effects, it can be understood as having a variety of productive consequences. For example, in so far as it is composed of relatively consistent assumptions, beliefs and concepts, a dominant approach can provide mental health professionals and those experiencing mental distress with an accessible way to comprehend and organise the sometimes complex, unusual and disturbing experiences that can be associated with such distress. Moreover, the tendency for one particular way of approaching mental distress to become dominant provides a common vocabulary or language that can be shared, understood and used by many. It further enables practitioners to coherently and efficiently communicate their clinical understandings with others and to consider, negotiate and determine their interventions on the basis of those shared understandings. However, despite its potentially productive effects, the fundamental danger associated with dominant ways of thinking and doing things in any field of human inquiry is that they can come to be understood as self-evident (Foucault 2002; Darder *et al.* 2017). That is, rather than being understood as a productive and yet provisional approach to human experience in which a variety of social, political and historical factors have contributed to its dominance, a favoured way of understanding and responding to any aspect of human experience, including mental distress, can come to be seen as obvious, unquestionable and even natural.

Once any one particular approach to mental distress comes to be held by an individual practitioner, a professional body or even an entire organisation as self-evident, then the opportunities to consider alternative ways of thinking and doing things can become significantly reduced. Indeed, when a dominant approach to mental distress comes to be accepted as obvious then, rather than being understood as resting upon assumptions and beliefs that are open to question, discussion and revision, it can come to be held as indisputable and therefore something which 'everybody knows' (Deleuze 2001, p. 130). Moreover, in so far as any approach comes to be accepted as self-evident, then the need to think and reflect critically about the particular way of understanding and responding to mental distress that it provides can not only seem unnecessary but it can even come to be dismissed as unreasonable. As Morgan (2006) suggests, however, when this occurs in any area of human inquiry then those dominant approaches or 'ways of seeing' that enable people to make sense of human experience and to negotiate that experience in an orderly way can become 'ways of not seeing' (p. 209). In particular, those favoured ways of thinking and doing things that enable a productive understanding and response to a certain feature of human experience, such as the experience of mental distress, can become constraints that prevent the consideration of alternative and potentially more productive ways of understanding and responding to that experience.

——————— CONCEPT SUMMARY: FORMS OF KNOWLEDGE ———————

Contemporary mental health care is informed by a diverse body of research, evidence and theory that originates from a variety of academic and clinical sources. However, following the distinction introduced by the German philosopher Jürgen Habermas (1972), mental health practice can be understood as requiring three distinguishable, and yet interconnected, forms of knowledge: technical knowledge, practical knowledge and emancipatory knowledge.

(Continued)

- **Technical knowledge** refers to the knowledge that is characteristic of the empirical sciences (such as biology, chemistry and physics) and is closely associated with evidence-based practice and technical health care interventions. In contemporary mental health care it can be understood as the knowledge that is required to decide, for example, the most effective psychotherapeutic techniques or psychiatric medication to use in response to a particular manifestation of mental distress.
- **Practical knowledge** refers to the knowledge that is associated with human interaction and which includes the skills necessary for effective interpersonal communication and mutual understanding to occur. In contemporary mental health care it can be understood as the knowledge that is required to develop therapeutic relationships with those experiencing mental distress as well as an awareness of the professional standards and values that characterise the development of those relationships.
- **Emancipatory knowledge** refers to the knowledge of those dominant ways of thinking and doing things in any sphere of human inquiry, and includes an awareness of how such dominance is maintained. In contemporary mental health care it can be understood as the knowledge that is required to engage critically with dominant approaches to mental distress and to participate in an exploration of potentially more productive ways of understanding and responding to that distress.

It is in the context of the tendency for certain ways of understanding and responding to mental distress to become dominant, and for those dominant approaches to come to be seen as obvious or natural, that we can understand the need for critical issues in mental health care. As you are probably already aware, rather than simply following instructions and getting things done without significant understanding and evaluation, as an autonomous and accountable mental health professional you are required to assess and justify the research, evidence and theory that informs the whole range of your clinical work. However, without an awareness of the critical issues raised by those who work within and those who use mental health services, your ability to assess your own practice, to examine how it may uncritically support supposedly self-evident ways of working, and to consider opportunities for practising in alternative and potentially more productive ways can be significantly diminished. For example, in highlighting the dangers that can accompany a failure to engage with alternative, critical perspectives in any area of human experience, and to reconsider the assumptions that underlie established approaches to that experience, Heath (2012) has suggested that 'If I only ever converse with people who agree with me, who share my assumptions and even my prejudices, I will not have access to the resources necessary to improve on my current levels of understanding' (p. 15).

Rather than having minimal significance for your practice, an engagement with critical issues in mental health care is therefore essential to becoming an informed, self-aware and proactive mental health professional. An awareness of these critical issues will not only provide you with the opportunity to begin to question approaches to mental distress that do not withstand critical examination, it will also enable a consideration of how to change those approaches as a result of contemporary research and evidence, the emergence of new theoretical perspectives and the active involvement and innovative work of those people who use mental health services. Moreover, in contrast to what have been referred to as 'superficial transformations', or changes that do not challenge dominant approaches to mental distress, a critical engagement with the assumptions that inform those approaches can produce the transformations in thought that are necessary to bring about productive transformations in practice. For example, while not underestimating the considerable challenges that are associated with questioning and seeking to change supposedly self-evident ways of thinking and doing things in any sphere of human inquiry, Foucault (1990) makes it clear that 'A transformation that remains within the same mode of thought … can merely be a superficial transformation. On the other hand, as soon as one can no longer think things as one formerly thought them, transformation becomes both very urgent, very difficult, and quite possible' (p. 155).

ACTIVITY 1.1   CRITICAL THINKING

Rather than being marginal to your mental health practice and being of academic interest only, an engagement with critical issues in mental health care is central to transforming your practice in ways that will make it more humane and responsive to the needs of those in distress.

For this activity critically consider how mental distress might still be understood, and what practices might still be in existence, if people in the past had not questioned, challenged and sought to change dominant and supposedly obvious ways of understanding and responding to that distress.

An outline answer is provided at the end of the chapter.

CRITICAL ISSUES AND INTELLECTUAL SKILLS

👥 CASE STUDY

Jonathan is currently at a two-day mental health conference and has just attended a presentation about the significance of critical issues for mental health professionals. In the presentation the speaker suggested that how practitioners understand and respond to mental distress is subject to ongoing critical examination, and those who use mental health services are demanding greater involvement in how their experiences are understood and addressed. Rather than simply accepting dominant and supposedly self-evident ways of working, the speaker argued that it is therefore becoming increasingly important for practitioners to 'engage actively' with

(Continued)

these critical developments and to consider them in the context of their own work. Reflecting upon the presentation afterwards, Jonathan is beginning to appreciate the importance of critical issues in mental health care for his own practice and for mental health services more generally. However, while he understands that this involves accessing reading material about contemporary critical issues, he is unsure how he should go about 'engaging actively' with those issues and what skills, dispositions or qualities such engagement requires.

To become a mental health professional who is able to consider critically and, where necessary, seek to change dominant and supposedly unquestionable ways of working, you will be required to possess more than a knowledge or an awareness of the critical issues that characterise mental health care. Indeed, it has been suggested that one of the most enduring and yet mistaken assumptions about the process of learning is that by simply acquiring knowledge a person will become an 'independent' or 'autonomous' thinker (Mezirow 1997). That is, it is commonly thought that by learning about a particular area of human inquiry, or gaining proficiency in the practical competencies that are associated with that area, a person will somehow spontaneously begin to question, challenge and even change its dominant and seemingly self-evident ways of thinking and doing things. In contrast to this assumption, the ability to become an informed and proactive mental health professional who is responsive to the needs of those who use mental health services not only requires an awareness of the critical issues that characterise contemporary mental health care; rather, it also necessitates an active engagement with those issues and a consideration of their significance in the context of your own professional practice. Like Jonathan in the above case study, however, it may not be immediately clear how to go about engaging actively with those issues and what skills, dispositions or qualities such an engagement demands.

An active engagement with the critical issues that can characterise any area of human inquiry, and the ability to challenge dominant ways of thinking and doing things as a result, requires the development of certain intellectual skills (Brookfield 2001; Paul & Elder 2014). A variety of intellectual skills have been proposed and you may already possess many if not all of these skills and be able to transfer them from other areas of your professional practice. In the context of mental health care, one of the most fundamental intellectual skills that is required to engage actively with critical issues is a willingness to ask, and be receptive to, questions about established and supposedly self-evident approaches to mental distress. While seemingly straightforward, this intellectual skill is closely associated with a variety of other 'habits of mind' in so far as it necessitates the ability to maintain a curiosity or inquisitiveness about existing ways of understanding and responding to mental distress, and, at least periodically, consider why things are the way they are. Irrespective of how developed your intellectual skills are, the ability to maintain a curiosity about the principles and practices that characterise mental health care will be central to an active engagement with critical issues because it is that which provides the disposition to ask and remain receptive to questions about dominant and supposedly obvious ways of working.

CONCEPT SUMMARY: INTELLECTUAL SKILLS

In order to acquire knowledge about any area of human inquiry, and to engage actively with the critical issues that can characterise that area, it is necessary to develop a variety of cognitive capabilities or intellectual skills (Bloom *et al.* 1956; Cottrell 2017). In the context of mental health care, a number of these intellectual skills can be understood as being of particular significance.

- **Comprehension** refers to the ability to understand the meaning or significance of the critical questions, debates and disputes that are a feature of contemporary mental health care. In particular, it requires an attempt to find ways of making sense of these issues even when they are experienced as being both personally and professionally challenging.
- **Application** is the ability to use our knowledge and understanding of a particular issue and employ it in a new situation. In doing so, it involves situating alternative approaches to mental distress in the context of our particular professional practice and considering the significance and relevance of those approaches in that unique context.
- **Synthesis** is the ability to bring seemingly separate elements together in order to form a new whole or create new meaning. It can involve making productive connections across the range of critical issues in mental health care in order to raise novel questions about, and consider alternatives to, existing approaches to mental distress.
- **Evaluation** refers to the ability to judge the quality of the evidence or arguments that are presented in support of a knowledge claim. In the process, it involves making an assessment about whether there are compelling reasons for understanding and responding to mental distress in a particular way or whether those reasons should be rejected.

As well as being challenging and contested, contemporary mental health care is also a complex area of professional practice. It has even been suggested that being a mental health professional 'inevitably involves us in some of the most important and perplexing questions that humans can face' (Kendler 2005, p. 439). While it can be tempting to simplify, disregard or even deny the complex character of the questions and debates that are a feature of mental health care, an active engagement with them will require you to confront and comprehend such complexity, and this, in turn, will require an ability to engage in analysis. As with many of the intellectual skills that can enable an active engagement with the principles and practices that characterise mental health care, analysis is a complex and multifaceted notion that has been defined in a variety of ways. However, to begin to understand what analysis means, it is instructive to recognise that its literal meaning is 'to loosen up' or 'to take things apart'. Therefore, in its most general sense, analysis can be understood as that intellectual activity which involves examining something in order to determine its constituent parts or the manner in which it is put together. In particular, analysis is commonly employed to examine something complex (which can be any theoretical or therapeutic feature of mental health care) in order to break it down into smaller elements and thereby clarify and deepen our understanding of that which has been taken apart.

While analysis involves examining something in order to determine its parts, and thereby comprehend its complexity, it is sometimes not immediately apparent how something in mental health care is put together. This is not only because the theoretical principles and therapeutic practices that help us to understand and respond to mental distress can be complex, but also because they can be composed of elements that are often implicit or hidden. In so far as they are ideas or beliefs that are assumed to be the case, these implicit elements or **assumptions** can profoundly influence how we think about and respond to mental distress and they commonly do so without our explicit awareness. Moreover, we inherit a wide range of assumptions from a variety of sources and they can often be maintained without good reason and be questionable, misinformed or even simply wrong. To engage actively with the complexity that can characterise critical issues in mental health care, and to consider the significance of those issues in the context of your own professional practice, the use of analysis will therefore not be limited to identifying the parts of something in order to comprehend such complexity. Rather, it will also involve attempting to 'unearth' or make explicit the variety of assumptions that can underlie any theoretical or therapeutic feature of mental health care in order to reflect upon the implications and appropriateness of maintaining those assumptions and, where necessary, consider their revision or even replacement.

ACTIVITY 1.2   TEAM WORKING

Rather than simply describing the world in a neutral and value-free manner, the language that we use is informed by a variety of assumptions that can be profoundly influential in producing, maintaining and changing how we understand and respond to the world (Bourdieu 1992; Foucault 2005; Fairclough 2015).

For this activity analyse the following terms that are, or have been, used in mental health care. As you do so, consider the assumptions or implicit ideas and beliefs that are associated with each term, and, with your colleagues, discuss the appropriateness of using them in the context of your professional practice.

- Mental illness;
- Mental health difficulty;
- Mental distress;
- Madness.

An outline answer is provided at the end of the chapter.

In addition to considering questions and conducting analyses, an active engagement with the critical issues that are a feature of contemporary mental health care requires an ability to reason. While reasoning is a multifaceted intellectual skill that has been defined and characterised in various ways, in its broadest terms it can be understood as identifying and evaluating the reasons given for something – whether that involves the reasons given for understanding something in a particular way or for doing something in a particular way (Fisher 2011). In the context of the dominance and supposedly self-evident nature of certain approaches to mental distress, however, it can be a particular challenge to identify the reasons that may underlie the use of such approaches. It may be that the reasons for understanding and responding to mental distress in a particular way are assumed to be obvious or, in addition to those that are given, you may suspect that there are other influential reasons that have been omitted. Alternatively, there may be a variety of reasons presented for why you should adopt one particular approach to mental distress as opposed to others, and the line or chain of reasoning may be long and complicated. For example, the reasons given for practising in a particular way might include formal or logical arguments, established or new research and evidence, theoretical orientations or philosophies, financial pressures or resource limitations, clinical experience or intuition and even appeals to authority or claims that 'this is the way it's always been done'.

Reasoning is not only used to determine what specific reasons are being given for understanding and responding to mental distress in a particular way. Rather, one of the primary aims of using reason in order to engage actively with critical issues in any area of human inquiry is to judge, or critically evaluate, the worth of those reasons (Swatridge 2014; Hanscomb 2017) – to judge, for example, whether the arguments, evidence or appeals to tradition that may be presented as reasons for adopting a particular theoretical and therapeutic approach to mental distress are convincing or whether they should be rejected as inconsistent, inconclusive or simply irrelevant. However, while it commonly involves evaluating the reasons of other individuals, professional bodies or entire organisations, a significant feature of reasoning is the ability to develop, clarify and articulate your own reasons. If you conclude that the reasons that are given for understanding and responding to mental distress in a particular way are not justified then you will need to articulate the reasons why you think that is the case. Moreover, if you think that the existing reasons given for practising in a particular way do not withstand critical evaluation, and that different ways of thinking and doing things in mental health care ought to be adopted, you will be required to make your reasons for such changes robust enough to withstand the questioning, analysis and reasoning of others.

CONCEPT SUMMARY: CRITICAL EVALUATION

Throughout your career as a mental health professional you will be introduced to a large amount of information that will form the various reasons given for why you ought to adopt a particular approach to mental distress. This will range from informal opinions, beliefs and

(Continued)

speculation to formal research, evidence and argument, and you will receive this information from a variety of sources, including lectures and tutorials, books and journal articles, presentations and conferences, professional guidance and peer discussions and, increasingly, through various forms of electronic media. Rather than simply accepting this information, it will be necessary to subject it to critical evaluation and to consider its value in the context of your professional practice. A variety of guidelines, methods and frameworks have been proposed to help you critically evaluate information and to critically appraise formal research in particular (Woolliams *et al.* 2011; Greenhalgh 2014). However, one of the most accessible and productive ways to critically evaluate the wide range of information that you will encounter as a mental health professional is to subject it to the following critically evaluative questions (Roberts 2015).

- **What does the information say?** This involves a consideration of the content of the information being presented and attempting to become clear about its meaning or position. While you may find that this is often a relatively straightforward process, on other occasions it can be more challenging and you may need to work hard, and use a variety of learning strategies, to clarify what is being said.
- **Where does the information come from?** This involves thinking about the source of the information and the extent to which it can be understood as credible. While it is possible to receive questionable information from reputable sources, and to obtain correct information from unreliable sources, finding out where it has come from can often provide you with a good indication of the quality of that information.
- **How has the information been produced?** The information that you will encounter as a mental health professional will have been produced through a variety of means, which can range from uninformed speculation to various sophisticated research methodologies. It can therefore be productive to assess the worth of those means and to consider if they are suitable for the particular area of mental health care being discussed.
- **Who has produced the information?** This involves an assessment of the experience and expertise of the individual or group that has produced the information. However, while it is important to respect the expertise of those who work within and use mental health services, it is necessary to focus upon the content of the information being presented without being overawed by, or dismissive of, those who have produced it.
- **Why has the information been produced?** This involves an attempt to determine the possible motives, interests and affiliations that may have influenced the production of a particular piece of information. In addition, it is necessary to consider if those motives, interests and affiliations have unduly influenced the production and presentation of the information in ways that are likely to misrepresent, mislead or even deceive others.
- **When was the information produced?** This involves thinking about whether the information is the best that is currently available and has not been superseded by more recent information. However, while discarding information on the basis of its age may be appropriate in relation to some areas of mental health care, doing so in other areas may unnecessarily restrict your discovery of potentially valuable information.

CRITICAL ISSUES AND EMOTIONAL QUALITIES

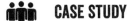 **CASE STUDY**

Amelia is a third-year student who is on her final clinical placement within a community mental health team before she qualifies as a mental health professional. She has quickly developed good relationships with the other practitioners and has discovered that many of them employ a cognitive behavioural approach to mental distress. Her mentor has told her that the team leader is a keen supporter of this approach and has worked hard to ensure almost all of the staff have attended some form of training course in cognitive behavioural therapy. Amelia is keen to develop her therapeutic skills in delivering this particular approach but has told her mentor that, as part of completing her practice assessment document, she is also required to display an understanding of a variety of approaches to mental distress. Her mentor has replied that while they can discuss these alternative approaches, they now have 'minimal relevance' in contemporary mental health care and, in thinking about her personal and professional development, she should focus upon developing her knowledge and skills surrounding cognitive behavioural therapy.

An active engagement with the questions and debates that can be a feature of any area of human inquiry is commonly characterised as an exclusively intellectual endeavour. As we highlighted at the beginning of this chapter, however, an engagement with critical issues in mental health care requires both the use of a variety of intellectual skills and the possession of a number of emotional qualities or dispositions. While you may already display many of these in the context of your professional practice, one of the most important emotional qualities for an awareness of and active engagement with critical issues in mental health care is an intellectual receptivity, or what is often referred to as an 'openness of mind'. While such a disposition is associated with a variety of other intellectual skills and emotional qualities (and, as in the case study above, can confront a number of obstacles) an openness of mind refers to a genuine and proactive willingness to consider new ideas, alternative perspectives and different ways of thinking and doing things (Hare 2007; Spiegel 2012). In the context of contemporary mental health care, open-mindedness requires us to become receptive to the critical issues that may challenge our favoured ways of understanding and responding to mental distress and, in the light of these challenges, to consider the possibility of thinking and working in alternative and potentially more productive ways.

CONCEPT SUMMARY: EMOTIONAL QUALITIES

While it is commonly characterised as a purely intellectual endeavour, there is a recognition that the emotions can assist us in gaining knowledge and actively engaging with the critical issues that can characterise any area of human inquiry (Hare 2011; Paul & Elder 2014). In the context

(Continued)

of contemporary mental health care, a number of these affective capabilities or emotional qualities can be understood as being of particular significance.

- **Honesty** is the disposition to acknowledge the possibility of having inconsistencies, biases and errors in our current understanding of, and response to, mental distress. Such an outlook requires us to uncover the various reasons why we may favour one particular approach to mental distress over others and to critically consider the legitimacy of those reasons.
- **Perseverance** is the quality of being determined to engage actively with critical issues in mental health care even when those issues are experienced as complex and challenging. It requires a commitment to continue to work through such complexities and challenges despite their potential to create various forms of personal and professional resistance.
- **Integrity** refers to the ability to be consistent when actively engaging with the critical issues that are a feature of mental health care. It requires us to hold ourselves, and our favoured ways of understanding and responding to mental distress, to the same rigorous standards of evidence and critical thought to which we hold others.
- **Humility** refers to an awareness of the limitations of our current knowledge and understanding. It involves not claiming to know more than we actually do about a particular issue and being willing to reconsider, revise and even reject our knowledge claims when confronted with compelling reasons to do so.

While an openness of mind requires a receptivity to alternative approaches to mental distress, it does not suggest an uncritical acceptance of any perspective and neither does it require you to treat all perspectives as being equally legitimate. In characterising open-mindedness as a 'hospitality' to new perspectives, Dewey (1980) memorably proposes that 'open-mindedness is not the same as empty-mindedness', it is not a hospitality that beckons 'Come right in; there is nobody at home' (p. 183). Rather, an active and considered engagement with critical issues in mental health care will require you to be cautious about readily accepting the latest perspectives and the 'buzz words' that can often accompany them, as well as being sceptical of those who claim to have established a definitive approach to mental distress. While it will require a receptiveness to new perspectives from a variety of sources, an openness of mind will therefore require you to subject those perspectives to critical evaluation and to consider their significance in the context of your own professional practice. In doing so, this critical receptivity can help prevent your practice from becoming limited by, and even 'entrenched' within, a single perspective. That is, an openness of mind can not only enable you to gain a deeper appreciation of the complexity of mental distress but it can also help to develop an awareness that critically considering different perspectives, and using a plurality of therapeutic approaches, will enable you to productively respond to the distress experienced by different people at different times.

CONCEPT SUMMARY: EGOCENTRISM

The notion of egocentrism has been used in a variety of disciplines and, in the context of child-hood cognitive development for example, refers to the manner in which young children have been characterised as being unable to distinguish their perspective from the perspective of others (Piaget 1959). However, egocentrism has been understood in broader terms as referring to the tendency of any person, irrespective of their age, to think and act exclusively from their own perspective without giving due consideration to alternative perspectives (Paul & Elder 2014). Moreover, while it can be a trait of an individual, it can also become manifest at the collective level, so that a group of people can embrace a particular perspective in such a way that the limitations of that perspective, and the strengths of other perspectives, are overlooked or even actively disregarded.

As one of the most common and yet profound obstacles to the development of our critical capabilities, egocentrism can be the result of a variety of powerful psychological processes. For example, rather than being justified by the available research, evidence and argument, we can support a particular way of understanding and responding to mental distress simply because it is the perspective we hold and thus we would like it to be true. In contrast, we can maintain a particular approach to mental distress because it is a perspective that we have uncritically adopted from others, such as the personal or professional group with which we associate. Alternatively, we can favour a particular way of working in mental health care, and actively disregard others, because it is in our vested interests to do so and it provides us with some form of personal, professional or financial reward.

In the context of the dominance and supposedly self-evident nature of certain ways of understanding and responding to mental distress, an openness of mind can be a particular challenge to develop and maintain. It is possible to form powerful and often biased attachments to particular approaches to mental distress and there can be a variety of personal, professional and organisational reasons, some of which might not be immediately apparent, why we may adhere to one particular approach without giving due consideration to others. An awareness of the ability to form emotional attachments to certain ways of thinking and doing things has led to the common suggestion that it is necessary to 'put aside' such attachments in order to somehow achieve a condition of 'pure rationality' and critical thought. However, rather than being a dispassionate and detached activity that is opposed to the influence of the emotions, the emotions can assist in learning about, and actively engaging with, critical issues in any area of human inquiry (Brookfield 2001; Reber 2016). Indeed, in the context of mental health care, an emotional engagement with the critical questions and debates which characterise that field of practice can be a powerful and productive force. It can not only motivate you to gain an awareness of those critical questions and debates, but it can also sustain your ongoing active consideration of them when confronted with a variety of obstacles, challenges and disincentives.

It is important to recognise, however, that simply possessing and displaying an emotional engagement with critical issues in mental health care is insufficient.

For example, an opposition to an existing way of understanding or responding to mental distress that is based solely on anger, no matter how intensely that emotion is felt, is unlikely to convince others of the merits of that opposition. Rather, in order to be considered a disciplined and fair-minded engagement with a critical issue, such emotional conviction will need to be accompanied by informed analysis, argument and reason. This does not mean that it is necessary to somehow achieve control or mastery over your emotions. Instead, an active engagement with critical issues in mental health care requires the development of an awareness of the power of the emotions both as a productive and non-productive influence on your thinking, along with a willingness to seek to harness the former influence while diminishing the latter. Such emotional self-awareness and management will therefore require a consideration of why you may favour certain approaches to mental distress over others, pursued with what may sometimes be experienced as an uncomfortable degree of honesty. You will be required to reflect, at least periodically, upon the reasons why you may be practising in certain ways and to think about whether doing so is justified by the available research, evidence and theory or whether it is a consequence of your emotional attachment to particular ways of working.

ACTIVITY 1.3   REFLECTION

Rather than being based upon the available research, evidence and theory, there may be a variety of alternative reasons why you favour one particular approach to mental distress over others. While it might not initially be clear to you what those reasons are, and while an investigation of them can produce varying degrees of personal resistance, for this activity reflect upon why you may support a certain approach to mental distress by considering the following questions.

- Do you maintain that approach as a result of 'intellectual complacency' and because that is the approach you have always adopted?
- Do you maintain that approach because it is shared by others, such as people in positions of authority or those whom you respect professionally?
- Do you maintain that approach because it is in your own self-interest to do so and because it provides you with some form of personal or professional advantage?

As this activity is based upon your own reflections, there is no outline answer at the end of the chapter.

In addition to open-mindedness and self-awareness, an emotional quality that is central to engaging actively with dominant and supposedly self-evident approaches to mental distress is courage. It may not be immediately clear why actively engaging with critical issues in mental health care requires courage until you remember that a fundamental feature of doing so is a willingness to raise and reflect upon a variety of questions about existing ways of understanding and responding to mental distress. Such engagement variously requires us to question our favoured ways of working in mental health care, to consider critically the legitimacy of the assumptions that underlie those ways of working and to reflect honestly upon the reasons why we may adopt one particular approach to mental distress over others. However, this can be a profoundly challenging process, both personally and professionally, and we ought not to underestimate how attached we can become to our favoured ways of thinking and doing things in mental health care. Indeed, as Brookfield (2001) makes clear, 'Asking critical questions about our previously accepted values, ideas, and behaviours is anxiety-producing. We may well feel fearful of the consequences that might arise from contemplating alternatives to our current ways of thinking and living'; at any stage of this process of questioning, challenging and considering changes to our existing ways of thinking and doing things, 'resistance, resentment, and confusion' can be evident (p. 7).

An active engagement with critical issues in mental health care can not only involve raising and reflecting upon challenging questions about our own ways of working, but it can also involve asking challenging questions about how others understand and respond to mental distress. Similar to the variety of reasons why we may be unwilling to question our favoured ways of working, there may be multiple reasons why other individuals, professional bodies and even entire organisations are reluctant to consider critically their particular approach to mental distress. As highlighted above, in the context of a health care culture that is focused on getting things done, and continually seeking to do so in the most efficient manner possible, an engagement with critical issues in mental health care can be perceived as a distraction or annoyance at best. At worst, however, such critical activity can be understood as a dangerous and subversive challenge to the aims and efficient functioning of the organisations in which mental health care is provided. While there will almost certainly be others within and beyond your immediate working environment who welcome the critical consideration of existing ways of working, and with whom you should seek to make productive alliances, there will be others who do not. The ability to question, challenge and potentially seek to change dominant and supposedly self-evident approaches to mental distress will therefore require you to display courage when faced with the individual, and sometimes even collective, resistance of others.

CHAPTER SUMMARY

This chapter has introduced you to the importance of critical issues in mental health care for your professional practice. It has suggested that an awareness of, and active engagement with, those issues will be fundamental to becoming an informed, self-aware and proactive mental health professional who is responsive to the needs of those who use mental health services. In particular, this chapter has suggested that the importance of such engagement can be understood in the context of the tendency for certain approaches to mental distress to become dominant and to be viewed as self-evident, unquestionable and even natural. Moreover, we have considered how an active engagement with the critical issues that characterise mental health care requires the development of a range of cognitive capabilities or intellectual skills. While various intellectual skills have been proposed, we have examined three that can be understood as being of particular significance: an ability to consider critical questions, to engage in analysis and to use the capacity to reason. While an engagement with critical issues in any area of human inquiry is commonly thought of as being a purely intellectual activity, this chapter has suggested that it also requires the possession of a number of affective capabilities or emotional qualities. While a variety of emotional qualities have been proposed, we have examined three that can be understood as being of particular significance for an engagement with critical issues in mental health care: an intellectual receptivity or openness of mind, an emotional self-awareness and management and, finally, the possession of courage.

ACTIVITIES: BRIEF OUTLINE ANSWERS

ACTIVITY 1.1 CRITICAL THINKING

There are a number of comprehensive, stimulating and controversial accounts of the history of mental distress and it will be productive to access and consider such accounts (Shorter 1997; Foucault 2001; Scull 2016). Importantly, when thinking about how mental distress has been understood in the past, and what practices were used to respond to such distress, you should be cautious about thinking of this history in terms of an unproblematic progression towards scientific and medical enlightenment. Multiple and competing histories have been written that illustrate how different approaches to mental distress sought to gain dominance at different times, with it being far from obvious which would prevail. However, you may have identified that in the past the experiences associated with mental distress were, for instance, understood in overtly religious terms. Viewed as being a consequence of the soul's possession by spirits and demons, or of God's vengeance for moral failings, a variety of spiritual means were used to respond to this perceived condition including prayer, pilgrimage or exorcism.

You may also have noted that while mental distress has been understood as possessing its own wisdom, during the 17th and 18th centuries it increasingly began to be thought of as a failure of reason and therefore to be understood in terms of 'irrationality'. In an attempt to 'shock' a person back to rationality a variety of interventions were used, such as whirling chairs and 'baths of surprise'. Moreover, you may have discussed with your colleagues the manner in which people who experienced mental distress in the past were confined in a variety of institutions, including private for-profit madhouses and public lunatic asylums. The quality of care provided in such institutions varied widely depending on a person's wealth, social status and family network, but, for the poor, life inside such institutions could be harsh. For example, you may have identified how a person inside such an institution could be subject to various forms of physical restraint including the use of chains, belts and straightjackets and multiple invasive physical interventions such as purges, vomiting and blood-letting.

ACTIVITY 1.2 TEAM WORKING

In analysing a number of terms that are, or have been, used in mental health care, and the appropriateness of using them in the context of your professional practice, you may have had complex and stimulating discussions with your colleagues. By analysing the assumptions or implicit ideas and beliefs that are associated with each term, you may have reflected upon how the language that is used to account for the experiences of those who use mental health services can profoundly influence how we understand and respond to those experiences. For example, you may have noted that the term mental illness is closely associated with a biological, or what is often referred to as a medical or biomedical, understanding of a person's experience. In contrast, mental health difficulty or mental health problem are often used as alternative terms in order to reflect a less biomedical understanding.

You might also have discussed how the term mental distress is increasingly favoured to emphasise each person's unique lived experience and to recognise the person that exists prior to any diagnostic category (NSUN 2015). Finally, in considering the term madness you may have discussed how it has been used to stigmatise, discriminate against and exclude those who use mental health services. However, you may also have identified that there have been attempts to reclaim the term by service user/survivor movements such as Mad Pride (Curtis *et al.* 2000). Similarly, while identifying the need to be cautious about using the term madness in the context of your practice because of its past pejorative connotations, you may have discussed how it is increasingly being used in some areas, such as **Mad Studies**, to challenge the theoretical and clinical assumptions associated with psychiatry (LeFrançois *et al.* 2013).

FURTHER READING

- **Cromby J, Harper D & Reavey P** (eds) (2013) *Psychology, Mental Health and Distress*. Basingstoke: Palgrave Macmillan.

This book provides a stimulating and sustained critical engagement with a range of critical questions, debates and disputes in contemporary mental health care, and does so in the context of various forms of mental distress.

- **Hall W** (ed) *Outside Mental Health: Voices and Visions of Madness*. Northampton, MA: Madness Radio.

A highly accessible collection of interviews and essays that cover a diverse range of critical issues about existing approaches to mental distress, with contributions from service users/survivors, mental health practitioners and academics.

- **Paul R & Elder L** (2014) *Critical Thinking: Tools for Taking Charge of Your Professional and Personal Life*, 2nd edition. New Jersey: Pearson Education.

This is an accessible work that discusses critical thinking in a personal and professional context as well as providing a sustained exploration of egocentrism and the range of emotional qualities that are associated with critical thinking.

- **Rapley M, Moncrieff J & Dillon J** (eds) (2011) *De-Medicalising Misery: Psychiatry, Psychology and the Human Condition*. Basingstoke: Palgrave Macmillan.

A thought-provoking book that provides various critiques of the theoretical and therapeutic features of contemporary mental health care conducted by those who work within, and those who have experience of using, mental health services.

USEFUL WEBSITES

- www.criticalpsychiatry.co.uk

Here you will find the website for the Critical Psychiatry Network, which provides a range of resources and articles that are concerned with questioning, challenging and seeking to change existing approaches to mental distress.

- www.criticalthinking.org

This is the website for the Centre for Critical Thinking, which provides a variety of resources about critical thinking, including how its development can be facilitated in educational settings and throughout society.

- www.madinamerica.com

Here you will find the website for Mad in America which provides information and education that seeks to challenge and explore alternatives to the dominance of drug-based approaches to mental distress in America and around the world.

- www.nationalelfservice.net/mental-health/

This is the website for The Mental Elf, which seeks to make evidence-based research in mental health care readily available to health and social care professionals and does so by providing short, accessible summaries of this research.

2

CAUSES OF MENTAL DISTRESS

CHAPTER AIMS

By the end of this chapter you will be able to:

* appraise the biological approach to mental distress;
* assess the trauma-informed approach to mental distress;
* examine the social and materialist approach to mental distress.

INTRODUCTION

👥 CASE STUDY

Over the past eight weeks, Kwame has become increasingly concerned about his fiancée Jessica. While ordinarily a sociable and active 22-year-old, Jessica has progressively stopped doing many of the things that she previously enjoyed and has instead been spending large amounts of the day and night sat silently in a chair by the dining room window. Moreover, while she normally has a healthy diet, she has been eating very little and Kwame has noticed that she appears to be losing weight. When asked about this, Jessica replies that there is something wrong with her digestive organs and this is preventing her from eating or drinking. Although Kwame has suggested that they should see someone to investigate this further she has replied that there is no point and, while she is somewhat vague about the details, has said that parts of her intestines are 'rotten' or are 'missing'. When Kwame attempts to clarify what she means, Jessica becomes agitated and irritable, insisting that she can no longer be helped and just wants to be left alone.

One of the most fundamental critical issues in contemporary mental health care is concerned with how to understand the causes of those experiences which can be associated with mental distress, experiences which can not only be unfamiliar but, as in the case study above, can be unexpected, confusing and disturbing. As you are probably already aware, the causes of mental distress have been understood by different societies and cultures in a variety of ways and competing histories have been written about how different approaches to mental distress came to replace and dominate others (Foucault 2001; Scull 2016). Moreover, in contrast to what have been referred to as **Whig histories** of psychiatry, in which debates about how to understand mental distress are presented as having been resolved (Shorter 1997; Lieberman 2016), the manner in which mental distress is conceptualised and thinking on what may contribute to its emergence and maintenance continue to be disputed. It is important to recognise, however, that such disputes are not detached from the everyday practice of contemporary mental health care. The explanatory framework that is employed to understand the causes of mental distress does not merely provide a particular perspective or a point of reference by which to organise and comprehend the experiences that are associated with such distress. Rather, each explanatory framework and the assumptions, beliefs and concepts of which it is composed profoundly influences what are considered to be the most appropriate interventions to employ in order to respond to those experiences.

The purpose of this chapter is therefore to introduce you to a variety of critical issues that are associated with how mental distress is understood and, in particular, with what contributes to the emergence and maintenance of that distress. It will begin by examining the approach that has variously been referred to as the biological, medical or biomedical model of mental distress, and which has been, and continues to be, vigorously debated by those who work within and those who use mental health services. In contrast to that model's assumption that mental distress is a manifestation of some form of biological dysfunction or disease process, and has no additional meaning or wider significance beyond such a process, this chapter will then discuss the emerging psychological and, in particular, trauma-informed approach to mental distress. In doing so, we shall consider how such distress can be understood as a meaningful response to traumatic and adverse events that can occur at various stages of an individual's life and especially during a person's childhood. Finally, within the context of the enduring assumption that the origin of mental distress is primarily to be found 'within' the individual – an assumption which has been associated with both biological and psychological approaches – this chapter will examine the social determinants of mental distress. In doing so, we shall consider how a range of social, economic and political factors that are located 'outside' or 'beyond' the individual, and which can profoundly influence and determine the social and material conditions of an individual's life, have been implicated in the emergence and maintenance of mental distress.

BIOLOGICAL APPROACHES TO MENTAL DISTRESS

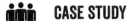 **CASE STUDY**

Adriana and her mental health colleagues are discussing the conditions that are conducive to recovery in the context of mental distress, and the ways in which they could be more concerned with the wider social context in which recovery occurs. In this context Adriana has suggested that it is necessary to develop strategies to address the multiple forms of **stigma**, prejudice and discrimination that service users/survivors often have to confront. For example, in order to begin to tackle such discrimination, she maintains that it is important for health care professionals and the wider public to become better educated about the causes of mental distress and to understand that such distress 'is an illness just like any other illness'. In particular, Adriana proposes that mental distress is commonly the result of biological dysfunctions and deficits which are beyond the control of the individual. Recognition of this fact should therefore enable people to understand that, rather than stigma, prejudice and discrimination, those who experience mental distress should be the recipients of care, compassion and respect.

Arguably the most influential and enduring way of understanding mental distress, as expressed by Adriana in the above case study, has been to view it as the manifestation of a disease process that has an underlying biological cause. In doing so, this understanding is also associated with the claim that the most appropriate and effective way of responding to such distress is through the use of various physical or biological interventions that supposedly address the disease processes or dysfunctions that are said to be the basis of mental distress. That this biological model has been profoundly influential can be discerned in the language that has characterised mental health care (e.g. mental 'illness', 'patients' and 'symptoms'), the people who have been deemed the most appropriate to provide that care (e.g. doctors, nurses and other 'health professionals') and the form of treatment that those who use mental health services are now most likely to receive (e.g. psychiatric drugs). Moreover, despite the emergence of a variety of alternative ways to understand and respond to mental distress, the biological model continues to have a powerful influence upon the work of many mental health professionals from a variety of disciplinary backgrounds. Indeed, while it is resisted by some, it has been suggested that the biological model also remains the approach that those who use mental health services often accept and 'internalise', at least initially, in order to comprehend the varied experiences associated with their mental distress (Cohen & Hughes 2011; Beresford *et al.* 2016).

While it is not exclusive to any one particular discipline, the biological model of mental distress has been most closely associated with psychiatry. Although it would be an oversimplification to maintain that it is the only model which informs that discipline, it has been suggested that psychiatry has made substantial efforts to determine an exclusively biological basis for mental distress in order to establish itself as a legitimate branch of medicine, somewhat similar to cardiology or neurology, that is concerned with identifying and treating biologically based medical disorders (Whitaker 2015; Scull 2016). In doing so, a variety of biological dysfunctions have been presented as being implicated in mental distress. For example, it has commonly been claimed that mental distress is a consequence of some form of 'chemical imbalance' and a deficiency or an over-stimulation of various neurotransmitters – the chemicals that are involved in the transmission of information between the neurons that make up the brain. It has also been claimed that behavioural and molecular genetic research has revealed that mental distress has a strong genetic component, with it also being proposed that particular genes are associated with certain forms of distress. Moreover, following the development of modern methods of imaging the living body – such as computerised axial tomography (CAT) and magnetic resonance imaging (MRI) – it has been suggested that various abnormalities with the structure and functioning of the brain are responsible for mental distress such as enlarged ventricles, grey matter loss in the cerebral cortex and brain-circuit dysfunction (Trimble & George 2010; Insel & Cuthbert 2015).

ACTIVITY 2.1   RESEARCH

It has been suggested that the various assumptions that underlie the modern biological approach to mental distress can be traced back to the 19th century and to the work of Emil Kraepelin (Bentall 2010; Hoff 2015).

For this activity conduct your own investigations into who Emil Kraepelin was and attempt to find out what contribution he made to the development of a biological approach to mental distress. An outline answer is provided at the end of the chapter.

Despite its enduring influence, the biological or biomedical model of mental distress continues to be subject to sustained criticism. Indeed, many of the critical issues in contemporary mental health care can be understood in terms of a response to, and often a rejection of, the principles and practices that are associated with this biological model. Arguably the most fundamental critique, however, is the suggestion that there is a lack of reliable, replicable and therefore compelling evidence for a clear biological cause in many forms of mental distress. With the exception of 'organic mental disorders' or 'organic brain syndromes' (such as Huntington's disease), it has been suggested that a clear and convincing biological cause has not been demonstrated for the vast majority of 'psychiatric disorders', including schizophrenia, bipolar disorder and depression (Cromby *et al.* 2013; Deacon 2013). For example, in what can be understood as a concise assessment of the attempt to establish an exclusively biological explanation for mental distress, Kenneth Kendler (2005) – a prominent researcher in the field of psychiatric genetics – has suggested that 'We have hunted for big, simple neuropathological explanations for psychiatric disorders and have not found them. We have hunted for big, simple neurochemical explanations for psychiatric disorders and have not found them. We have hunted for big, simple genetic explanations for psychiatric disorders and have not found them' (pp. 434–435).

CONCEPT SUMMARY: THE EQUAL ENVIRONMENT ASSUMPTION

Among the variety of research methods used to support the claim that schizophrenia is a highly heritable genetic condition, the most frequently used is said to be the classical twin method. This method compares the prevalence of a diagnosis of schizophrenia in identical twins (twins which develop from one fertilised egg cell) and who have been reared together, with the prevalence of a diagnosis of schizophrenia in same sex, non-identical twins (twins which develop from two fertilised egg cells) and who have been reared together. In doing so, it is assumed that the identical and non-identical twins are exposed to equally similar environments such that any difference in the rates of schizophrenia between identical and non-identical twins is therefore attributable to genetic factors. However, this equal environment assumption, an assumption which underlies the classical twin method, has been subject to sustained critique.

In particular, it has been suggested that rather than being equal, the environments of identical and non-identical twins are significantly different with identical twins more likely to be dressed the same, to spend more time together, to have common friends and to be treated differently by others (Joseph 2013, 2015). Importantly, it has also been claimed that identical twins are more likely to be exposed to a range of environmental factors (including childhood trauma) that have been associated with the emergence and maintenance of those distressing experiences associated with a diagnosis of schizophrenia (Fosse *et al.* 2015). It has therefore been argued that the classical twin method does not adequately disentangle the potential influence of genes and environment when considering the causes of schizophrenia and, as such, cannot provide a valid indication of genetic effects in that form of mental distress (Fosse *et al.* 2016).

To suggest that there is no compelling evidence for a clear biological cause in many forms of mental distress may strike some as a challenging and controversial claim, especially in the context of assertions in the mass media and the health care literature of breakthroughs and revolutions in the biological understanding of mental distress (Insel 2015; Lieberman 2016). However, when such findings are subsequently examined in detail it is not uncommon for them to be characterised by various unwarranted assumptions, logical flaws and methodological problems, such that 'often, an initial proclamation of success is followed, sometime later, by a much less publicized failure to replicate initially promising findings' (Cromby *et al.* 2013, p. 78). Moreover, where biological differences have been found between those who have experienced mental distress and those who have not, the challenge has been to demonstrate the significance of these differences and this challenge, it is claimed, has yet to be met. That is, it is necessary to demonstrate the pathways, processes and mechanisms by which those biological differences can lead to the range of experiences that are associated with various forms of mental distress, rather than such differences being a consequence of, for example, various environmental factors, the confounding effects of psychiatric treatment or the experience of mental distress itself (Read & Bentall 2013; Kendler 2014).

CONCEPT SUMMARY: THE CONFOUNDING EFFECTS OF PSYCHIATRIC DRUGS

One of the most enduring biological explanations for mental distress is the dopamine hypothesis of schizophrenia, in which it is suggested that the distressing experiences associated with a diagnosis of schizophrenia, and psychosis in general, are a consequence of a biochemical abnormality with the neurotransmitter dopamine. In particular, findings from post-mortem studies on the brain tissue of those with a diagnosis of schizophrenia led to the suggestion that an over-abundance of dopamine receptors may be responsible for the emergence and maintenance of that form of mental distress (Lee & Seeman 1980).

Subsequent research indicated, however, that the increase in dopamine receptors was only detected in those who had received long-term treatment with anti-psychotic drugs (Mackay *et al.* 1982; Kornhuber *et al.* 1989). Therefore, rather than being a biological abnormality that caused schizophrenia, it was concluded that the over-abundance of dopamine was a consequence or confounding effect of the use of anti-psychotic drugs. In particular, this over-abundance was said to be the result of the brain's attempt to compensate for how those drugs inhibit the action of dopamine (Moncrieff 2008; Whitaker 2015).

More recently, the detection of other differences in the brains of those with a diagnosis of schizophrenia, differences which might initially seem to indicate a possible biological explanation for that form of mental distress, have been said to be a consequence of the use of anti-psychotic drugs. While such findings remain controversial (Roiz-Santianez *et al.* 2015), it has been suggested that those drugs may produce a variety of significant 'neuroanatomical alterations', such as grey matter loss, white matter loss and enlarged ventricles (Ho *et al.* 2011; Fusar-Poli *et al.* 2013).

To suggest that there is as yet no compelling evidence for an exclusively biological cause of mental distress is not to propose that biology is insignificant for an understanding of the experience or causes of mental distress. All of our experiences are dependent upon, enabled by and expressed within our biological systems – a state of embodiment which it has been suggested is sometimes neglected by those seeking to provide alternatives to the biological model (Boyle 2015). However, there is a growing recognition that the varied experiences that are associated with mental distress cannot satisfactorily be reduced to, and fully explained by, human biology, and it should therefore not possess the primary or foundational role that is given to it by the biological model of mental distress. As a consequence of conceptual and empirical work in a number of disciplines (such as **developmental neuroscience** and **epigenetics**), more sophisticated models of mental distress are beginning to emerge in which both biology and environmental factors are understood as being in a continuous and reciprocal relationship (Schore 2005; Read *et al.* 2014; Nestler *et al.* 2016). Such understandings propose that the causes of mental distress cannot be explained exclusively in terms of biology and neither can they be explained exclusively in terms of the environment. Rather, in moving beyond having to make a dichotomous choice between nature or nurture, these emerging models propose that mental distress must be understood in terms of the irreducible, interdependent and dynamic relationship between the two.

——— CONCEPT SUMMARY: MODERN ATTACHMENT THEORY ———

By combining the insights of developmental neuroscience, child psychiatry and John Bowlby's (1969) theory of attachment, modern attachment theory (or what is also referred to as regulation theory) maintains that mental distress is a consequence of the relationship between an individual's biology and their environment (Schore & Schore 2008). In particular, it suggests that while the rapid growth of an infant's brain during the first 18 months is partially encoded by the individual's **genome**, brain development (and specifically those regions of the right hemisphere that are associated with the regulation of emotion, the establishment of relationships and a coherent sense of self) is also 'shaped indelibly' by the emotional communications that characterise the attachment relationship between a child and its primary caregiver (Schore 2005).

While a secure attachment relationship is said to create the conditions for optimal neurobiological and psychosocial growth, a 'disorganised' or 'disorientated' attachment relationship (which can be associated with traumatic and adverse events) can have lasting detrimental effects upon the area of the brain involved in emotional self-regulation, which, it is argued, can provide the basis for the development of mental distress in later life (Schore 2001). Therefore, modern attachment theory does not attempt to reduce the origin of mental distress to either biology or the environment, but proposes that its emergence can be a consequence of the interdependent and dynamic interaction between the individual's genetic disposition and the social-emotional environment in which that individual is situated during infancy.

If there is no compelling evidence for an exclusively biological cause of mental distress, the question arises as to how such an understanding has maintained its authoritative influence in mental health care. As highlighted in the previous chapter, the reasons why any one particular approach to mental distress gains precedence are complex and contested and a variety of critical reasons for the emergence and continuing influence of the biological model have been proposed, reasons which have little to do with its supposed theoretical and therapeutic superiority over other approaches to mental distress (Boyle 2015; Busfield 2015; Whitaker & Cosgrove 2015). For example, it has been suggested that the pharmaceutical industry contributes to the continued influence of the biological model in a variety of ways, such as through the misrepresentation of research data that claims to establish the biological basis of mental distress and the effectiveness of psychiatric drugs to respond to that distress. In addition, the influence of the biological model has been attributed to a societal tendency, supported by the mass media, to favour biological and individualistic accounts of mental distress, along with a deference towards the medical profession and a reluctance to question medical explanations. Moreover, it has been proposed that the ongoing influence of the biological model can be attributed to the employment of a whole range of questionable strategies that are used by individuals, groups and even entire organisations to marginalise, delegitimise and exclude alternative ways of understanding and responding to mental distress.

———— CONCEPT SUMMARY: THE BIOPSYCHOSOCIAL MODEL ————

One of the most effective ways in which the biological model of mental distress is said to have maintained its influence, especially while being subject to sustained critique, is by assimilating alternative perspectives and removing or neutralising the critical considerations associated with those perspectives. Such a process can be discerned in particular conceptions of the biopsychosocial model of mental distress, a model which supposedly integrates biological, psychological and social factors as equally important in understanding the causes of such distress (Engel 1977).

However, rather than maintaining their equal, irreducible and reciprocal relationship, it has been suggested that the biopsychosocial model gives primacy to the influence of biological factors in the emergence and maintenance of mental stress. In particular, by drawing on the notion of **stress-vulnerability** (Zubin & Spring 1977), the biopsychosocial model is said to commonly present psychological and social factors as the stressors that 'trigger' a supposedly more fundamental biological, and in particular genetic, vulnerability to mental distress (Boyle 2015).

While this understanding of the biopsychosocial model acknowledges the influence of psychological and social factors, they are of secondary importance in comparison with the biological vulnerability that supposedly underlies mental distress. Indeed, in highlighting how such an understanding perpetuates the authoritative influence and privileged status of the biological approach to mental distress, Read (2005) has suggested that the biopsychosocial model of mental distress 'is not an integration of models, it is a colonisation of the psychological and social by the biological' (p. 597).

TRAUMA-INFORMED APPROACHES TO MENTAL DISTRESS

One of the most fundamental assumptions of an exclusively biological approach to mental distress is that the various experiences that can be associated with such distress, including hearing voices or having unusual beliefs, are meaningless and therefore not understandable. That is, in so far as the biological model maintains that mental distress is a consequence of some form of biological dysfunction then the experiences which can be associated with such distress are understood to be the outward manifestations of an underlying disease process, and, as such, they do not possess any additional meaning or wider significance beyond such a process. Indeed, it has even been suggested that the attempt to seek a wider significance in mental distress is an inappropriate, misguided and ultimately unscientific endeavour that is incompatible with attempts to establish psychiatry as a legitimate branch of medicine that identifies and treats biologically based medical disorders (Insel 2009; Lieberman 2016). However, understanding the experiences associated with mental distress as a meaningless manifestation of an underlying disease process has potentially profound implications for the practice of mental health professionals. For example, in highlighting these consequences, Johnstone (2008, p. 13) has concisely concluded that:

> If hearing voices, or being low in mood, or intensely anxious, or fearing that you are being poisoned by your relatives, are diagnosed as the 'symptoms' of an 'illness', there is no more reason for professionals to enquire into them than into the meaning of a rash, or the content of delirious speech in a fever.

The assumption that mental distress is meaningless has periodically been challenged from a variety of psychiatric, psychological and philosophical perspectives (May 1950; Laing 1960). In contemporary mental health care, this challenge can be seen in the emerging body of research that has investigated the ways in which mental distress can be understood as a meaningful response to trauma – where trauma refers to events or situations that are experienced as harmful, violent and life-threatening and which are often associated with overwhelming feelings of terror, horror and helplessness (Herman 2015; Sweeney *et al.* 2016). Trauma at various stages of an individual's life has been implicated in the aetiology of mental distress, including those experiences associated with a diagnosis of post-traumatic stress disorder. However, particular emphasis has been placed on the relationship between mental distress in adulthood and a range of traumatic and adverse events that can occur in childhood, including parental death, witnessing violence at home, and physical, sexual and/or emotional abuse (Kessler *et al.* 2010). It is important to recognise that childhood trauma is not only a significant risk factor for those experiences associated with a diagnosis of, for example, depression, anxiety and eating disorders, but it is has also been suggested that it is 'substantially associated' with an increased risk of psychosis and those experiences, such as hearing voices and unusual beliefs, that have often been understood as the meaningless outward manifestation of an underlying biological dysfunction (Varese *et al.* 2012; Bentall *et al.* 2014; Palmier-Claus *et al.* 2016).

👤👤👤 CASE STUDY

Now in his early forties, Steven first became involved with mental health services over twenty years ago when he began to experience disturbances in his mood and thoughts that were also associated with hearing voices. He was subsequently given a diagnosis of schizophrenia and has since had multiple mental health hospital admissions, the most recent coinciding with the

(Continued)

death of his father just over six months ago. While he now rarely reflects upon what may have contributed to his mental distress, Steven initially thought that it may have been related to a number of traumatic events that occurred during his childhood. Following one of his earliest admissions to hospital he can recall alluding to these childhood events with a mental health professional and attempting to discuss their potential significance. However, he also remembers receiving the impression that doing so made the other person 'uncomfortable' and he was informed that, while undoubtedly distressing at the time, those past events were unlikely to have had a significant bearing upon the development and maintenance of his symptoms.

ACTIVITY 2.2   TEAM WORKING

The suggestion that traumatic and adverse events in childhood are a significant risk factor for many forms of mental distress, including psychosis, continues to be a controversial claim in contemporary mental health care. Moreover, it has been suggested that 'Mental health professions have been slow, even resistant, to recognise the role of childhood adversities in psychiatric disorder' (Read & Bentall 2012, p. 89).

For this activity discuss with your colleagues why you think investigations into the relationship between childhood trauma and adult mental distress have been, and continue to be, controversial. As you do so, attempt to explain why mental health professionals, as illustrated by Steven's experience in the above case study, may be reluctant to recognise and respond to this relationship.

An outline answer is provided at the end of the chapter.

To propose that traumatic events in childhood can contribute to mental distress in later life is not to claim that every adult who experiences mental distress has been subject to childhood trauma, and neither is it to claim that every child who has experienced trauma will necessarily develop clinical levels of mental distress. The reasons why those who have a history of childhood trauma will have different outcomes with respect to the forms and the severity of mental distress that they experience will be influenced by a variety of factors. For example, such outcomes can be influenced by whether a child blames themselves for the trauma, the resources they have to respond to its effects and the presence of supportive social networks and safe attachment figures (Barker-Collo & Read 2003). There is also an emerging body of research highlighting the complex relationship between childhood trauma and the developing brain. As discussed above in the context of modern attachment theory, this research is being used to develop more sophisticated models of how the relationship between a child's environment and their neurobiological development can contribute to mental distress in later life. Such models maintain that instead of being reducible to either the individual's biology or their environment (and rather than simply treating environmental factors such as childhood trauma as stressors that trigger a supposedly more fundamental biological vulnerability), the development of mental distress should be understood in terms of the interdependent and reciprocal relationship between the two (Read *et al.* 2014).

The emerging recognition of the role of childhood trauma in the development of mental distress in later life highlights the importance of situating that distress within the context of an individual's life and reflecting upon how it may be a meaningful response to a range of adversities (Dillon 2010). Indeed, there is evidence to suggest that the content of those experiences that are associated with psychosis and which have often been taken to be the meaningless manifestation of an underlying disease process can be understood in the biographical context of a person's life. In particular, it has been claimed that the content of a person's voice-hearing experience can have varying degrees of correspondence with the childhood adversities to which that person may have been subject (Reiff *et al.* 2012; Corstens & Longden 2013). Moreover, even where there does not appear to be a direct relationship between a person's voice-hearing experience and childhood trauma, it is possible to develop a joint formulation or **construct** in which that experience can be understood as meaningful. In particular, it has been suggested that the content of a person's voice-hearing experience can variously be understood as a representation of significant figures in that individual's life or an expression of dissociated aspects of that individual's self or personality, as well as an embodiment of the emotional conflict that has resulted from the trauma that the person may have experienced during childhood (Longden *et al.* 2012).

CONCEPT SUMMARY: THE INTERNATIONAL HEARING VOICES MOVEMENT

Influenced by the work of Marius Romme and Sandra Escher (1993, 2000), the hearing voices movement is an international collective that seeks to enable people to accept and understand the experience of hearing voices in the unique context of their life (Corstens *et al.* 2014). Rather than being understood as the meaningless 'symptom' of a 'mental illness' that is to be denied or suppressed by a variety of means, the hearing voices movement maintains that voice hearing is a normal human variation.

In doing so, this movement distances itself from terminology, such as 'auditory hallucinations', that is associated with a biomedical and predominately pathologising approach to the voice-hearing experience. While acknowledging that it can be profoundly disturbing, the experience of hearing voices is instead understood as something which can be a meaningful expression of distressing experiences in a person's life and the emotional conflicts that have arisen as a result of those experiences.

In maintaining that voice hearing can be meaningful, the hearing voices movement does not promote any one interpretation or explanatory frame of reference to account for that experience. Rather, by prioritising the subjective reality of the individual, it seeks to encourage each person (often in peer support meetings known as 'hearing voices groups') to develop their own understanding of, and ways of coping with, that experience, and even to find within it the potential for new meaning and personal development.

As a consequence of the increasing awareness of the manner in which trauma at various stages of an individual's life can contribute to mental distress, it has been suggested that there is a need for a trauma-informed transformation of contemporary mental health care (Sweeney et al. 2016). However, rather than only seeking to facilitate change in the knowledge, values and skills of individual practitioners, such an approach is also said to require a comprehensive and potentially challenging cultural transformation of the organisations in which those practitioners are situated (Bloom & Farragher 2013). This cultural transformation requires the development of a greater awareness of the manner in which mental distress can arise as a meaningful response to adverse events rather than being understood, for example, as a manifestation of some form of biological or psychological dysfunction. It has therefore been suggested that trauma-informed approaches in mental health care require a 'vital paradigm shift' from the prevailing attempt to determine 'what is wrong with a person', and should instead be concerned with asking 'what has happened to this person' (Harris & Fallot 2001; Longden 2010). Such a transformation will not only require training, supervision and support for all mental health professionals to develop the ability to decide when and how to inquire about whether a person has been subject to trauma; rather, it will also demand the provision of trauma-specific interventions for those who require them and the development of clear pathways to enable people who use mental health services to access those interventions (Read et al. 2007).

In recognising that those who use mental health services may have been subject to trauma and adverse events, trauma-informed approaches to mental distress require a thoroughgoing commitment to cause no further harm (Filson 2016). In particular, there is a need for a greater awareness of, and responsiveness to, the variety of ways in which mental health services can potentially re-traumatise an individual. This can occur following an incident in the present that is reminiscent of a past traumatic incident and which can elicit the same or similar physiological, psychological and behavioural responses that were associated with that past event. As such, there is an understanding that those who use mental health services can be re-traumatised through witnessing or being subject to a range of traumatic events that can occur in mental health settings, such as physical restraint, the use of seclusion, threats of enforced detention and unwanted sexual advances (Frueh et al. 2005). In creating therapeutic environments that cause no further harm and promote the safety of those who use mental health services (where safety is understood in physical, psychological and emotional terms) the trauma-informed transformation of mental health care therefore requires a commitment to non-violence. This not only involves the reduction and even elimination of practices such as seclusion, restraint and forced medication, it also requires the eradication of the multiple **microaggressions** to which service users/survivors can be subject, including demeaning and infantilising language, subtle forms of coercion and the marginalisation of a person's understanding of their mental distress (Bloom & Farragher 2013; Gonzales et al. 2015).

SOCIAL APPROACHES TO MENTAL DISTRESS

Alongside the notion that mental distress is meaningless, one of the most enduring assumptions associated with a biological approach to mental distress is that the origin of that distress is to be found within the individual, a consequence of some form of individual biological dysfunction. However, this individualistic assumption is not exclusive to a biological approach to mental distress, but (as we shall discuss in detail in Chapter 5) can be understood as being characteristic of the theory and practice of various psychological and psychotherapeutic approaches to mental distress (Boyle 2011; Smail 2014). Indeed, rather than being exclusively associated with either a biological or a psychological approach, it has been suggested that the location of the origin of mental distress within the individual is characteristic of the **technological model of mental distress** that has come to dominate contemporary mental health care. As highlighted in the previous chapter, this dominant approach to mental distress is said to be largely individualistic in so far as it understands that distress as primarily having its origin within the individual, a manifestation of some form of underlying biological or psychological dysfunction. In doing so, it also maintains that the most appropriate way to respond to mental distress is by seeking to transform the individual's thoughts, feelings and behaviours through the expert application of various forms of technical intervention such as psychiatric drugs or cognitive behavioural therapy (Bracken *et al.* 2012; Coles *et al.* 2015).

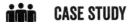 **CASE STUDY**

Samira is a 25-year-old single woman with a four-year-old daughter who has been attempting to fund herself through university by working in a bar in the evening. However, she has recently been made redundant from that job and, despite making numerous inquiries and applications, has so far been unable to find alternative employment. As a consequence Samira has been experiencing significant financial difficulties and has been struggling to meet the expense of feeding herself and her daughter – which she has so far been able to do by reducing the use of heating in her flat. While she has been surviving on the small amount of money that she had managed to save over the past 18 months, she is becoming increasingly concerned and anxious about her financial situation. These concerns have been made worse by ongoing disputes and delays with the local authority about the amount of financial assistance to which she is entitled. As a consequence, she has not only begun to feel increasingly isolated with her current difficulties, but is starting to feel helpless about being able to resolve those difficulties.

As with the notion that mental distress is meaningless, the assumption that the origin of such distress is primarily located within the individual has periodically been challenged from a variety of political, sociological and philosophical perspectives (Fromm 1955; Laing 1967). It has thus been suggested that while mental distress finds its expression within or 'through' the individual, a multiplicity of factors that are located 'outside' or 'beyond' the individual may be more significant when considering the origins of the emergence and maintenance of that distress. Indeed, the manner in which mental distress has been presented as a meaningful response to trauma entails that, rather than being reducible to some form of individual dysfunction, such distress can be understood in interpersonal terms and within the context of the adverse interpersonal relationships and conditions to which a person can be subject. However, the assumption that the origin of mental distress is to be found within the individual has also been challenged by research into the manner in which it can be associated with a variety of broader social, economic and political factors to which an individual may be exposed. As illustrated in the above case study, these socio-economic factors or social determinants can profoundly influence and determine the social and material conditions of people's lives and, in doing so, increase the possibility of the emergence and maintenance of mental distress throughout the course of those lives (Compton & Shim 2015).

CONCEPT SUMMARY: NEOLIBERALISM

The enduring assumption that the origin of mental distress is primarily located within the individual, a consequence of some form of biological dysfunction or psychological deficit, can be understood as a reflection of the neoliberal conception of being human that has become dominant throughout contemporary Western societies. Although a multifaceted concept, in its broadest terms **neoliberalism** refers to a political and economic ideology that, while having its origins in 18th-century thought, was reinvigorated at the end of the 20th century and has since become the dominant ideology of many societies around the world. As a collection of political and economic practices, neoliberalism is associated with the de-regulation or 'liberalisation' of finance, trade and markets, the erosion of trade union representation, and the privatisation of public services such as energy, transport and health (Harvey 2007).

It is in this context that neoliberalism conceptualises human beings in individualistic or 'atomistic' terms and maintains that people prosper when, in competition with others, they pursue their own self-interests and draw upon their own resources to secure those interests (Springer 2016). In order to facilitate this, neoliberalism advocates a reduction in state intervention and public expenditure, such that the obligation of governments to provide for the welfare of a country's citizens is progressively diminished. In doing so, neoliberalism is associated with an ethic of self-reliance, independence and personal responsibility. With a sufficient amount of 'hard work' and 'will power' the individual is often presented as being able to overcome any social and material disadvantage, while the hardships and distress that people do undergo are commonly characterised as some form of personal failing, weakness or deficiency.

ACTIVITY 2.3   RESEARCH

The individualistic orientation of contemporary mental health care, and the notion that mental distress is a consequence of some form of biological or psychological dysfunction, can be understood as a reflection of the individualistic conception of being human that characterises neoliberalism.

In considering how a variety of social determinants may contribute to mental distress, it can therefore be productive to investigate alternative ways of understanding human beings which emphasise how each person is embedded within, and influenced by, a variety of social systems.

For this activity conduct your own research into Urie Bronfenbrenner's (1979) 'ecological systems theory'. In particular, summarise how it understands the relationship between human beings and the social environment and how this can help to understand the influence of social factors on mental distress.

An outline answer is provided at the end of the chapter.

Given their complex, interdependent and dynamic character, it can be a considerable challenge to understand the variety of social determinants to which a person can be subject and the manner in which those determinants may contribute to the emergence and maintenance of mental distress. In making a start, however, it is productive to recognise the spatial metaphor that is commonly used to make a distinction between proximal and distal social determinants and to distinguish the diversity of such determinants in particular (Smail 2014). Accordingly, **proximal social determinants** are those social factors which have a 'close proximity' to an individual and can therefore exert their influence upon a person's mental health from a comparatively 'short distance' and in a direct and immediate way. Such proximal social determinants include unemployment or low-paid, insecure employment; poor housing, insecure living conditions and homelessness; and low-quality neighbourhoods with multiple social stressors such as vandalism, noise pollution and crime. In contrast, **distal social determinants** are those social factors which exist 'farther away' from an individual and therefore exert their influence from a 'greater distance' and often in an indirect, delayed manner through a variety of other mediating factors. Such distal social determinants include local and national decisions on health and welfare expenditure, the availability of affordable housing, policing levels and migration policies, as well as the occurrence of economic recessions and the levels of wealth inequality throughout society.

Rather than locating the origin of mental distress within the individual, investigations into the social determinants of mental health can therefore be understood as shifting the focus of concern onto how those determinants – and social inequality, disadvantage and injustice more generally – can contribute to mental distress. In doing so, there is a significant body of research to indicate that the prevalence of mental distress is more common in more unequal societies. In particular, an increase in wealth inequality, and in the gap between the richest and the poorest members of society, is not only associated with an increase in 'common' forms of mental distress such as depression, anxiety and substance misuse, but also with 'severe' forms of mental distress such as psychosis (Wilkinson & Pickett 2010; Kirkbride *et al.* 2014; WHO 2014). However, the association between wealth inequality and mental distress is not simply attributable to the ongoing challenge of having to deal with the consequences of social and material disadvantage, nor to the likelihood of having fewer material resources to be able to absorb and alleviate the occurrence and consequences of challenging life events; rather, it has been suggested that the association is also attributable to the way in which wealth inequality, as a distal social determinant, is closely related to a number of proximal social determinants that can increase the risk of mental distress, such as unemployment or insecure employment, poor housing and insecure living conditions, as well as traumatic and adverse events in childhood (Read & Bentall 2013; Rogers & Pilgrim 2014).

CONCEPT SUMMARY: ECONOMIC RECESSION AND MENTAL DISTRESS

An economic recession is a significant reduction in activity across a country's economy that is commonly defined as a decline in **gross domestic product** for at least two consecutive quarters, where a quarter is equivalent to three months. Such economic events commonly lead to a reduction in the manufacture and sale of goods, a decline in business profits and an increase in the rate of unemployment, as well as a reduction in household incomes and a fall in consumer demand for products and services. While they have far-reaching effects across a country's economy, economic recessions also have significant consequences for the mental health of citizens. These include an increase in various forms of mental distress such as depression and anxiety, a rise in the misuse of alcohol and drugs and an increase in the rates of suicide, particularly in males of working age (Chang *et al.* 2013).

The precise ways in which economic recessions can contribute to mental distress is a matter of ongoing critical consideration. However, it has been suggested that the events and conditions that recessions can produce (such as unemployment, financial difficulties, home repossession and marital conflict) can create a sense of insecurity, hopelessness and worthlessness, and this can contribute to anxiety, substance misuse, depression and an increased risk of suicide. Moreover, it has also been proposed that the response of governments to engage in austerity measures at a time of economic recession (such as cuts to health and welfare expenditure) can further intensify the hardships experienced by the most disadvantaged in society, and this can be an additional contributory factor in the development and maintenance of mental distress for those people (Van Hal 2015; Haw *et al.* 2016).

While the research into the social determinants of mental health highlights a clear association between social inequality and mental distress, the reasons for that relationship have been contested. In particular, it has been suggested that social inequality and, for example, unemployment, poor living conditions and impoverished circumstances do not cause mental distress. Rather, it has been argued that a person is more likely to move or 'drift' down the social scale and into insecure unemployment, poor living conditions and impoverished circumstances as a result of their pre-existing mental health problems. However, this social drift hypothesis has been critiqued from a variety of perspectives. Not only has it been suggested that the evidence for such an explanation is poor, but it has also been argued that it serves to neutralise the critical force of alternative perspectives and perpetuate the individualistic orientation of the principles and practices that characterise contemporary mental health care (Boyle 2011). That is, by suggesting that mental distress causes social inequality rather than being a consequence of that inequality, the social drift hypotheses can be used to support the assumption that the origin of that distress is to be found within the individual. Indeed, even where the social drift hypothesis acknowledges that social factors can contribute to mental distress, it relegates those factors to stressors that trigger an individual's supposedly pre-existing biological or psychological vulnerability to such distress.

As with the biological and trauma-informed approaches to mental distress, however, the attempt to determine the precise pathways, processes and mechanisms by which social determinants can contribute to the emergence and maintenance of such distress can be an extraordinarily complex endeavour (Shah *et al.* 2011). Rather than seeking to definitively determine whether social inequality can cause mental distress or whether such inequality is a consequence of that distress, it has been suggested that 'circular relationships, rather than linear ones, capture the relationship between the social and the mental health of persons and render older arguments about social stress and downward drift as futile' (Pilgrim & Rogers 2008, p. 24). Therefore, while it is important to recognise that mental distress can contribute to social inequality, and while it is equally important to recognise that social inequality can contribute to mental distress, the complex relationship between the two means that the attempt to prioritise one over the other is overly simplistic. Instead, it has been suggested that a more sophisticated and complete analysis of the relationship between social inequality and mental distress ought to recognise the importance of, and consider how best to respond to, the manner in which mental distress can be both a cause and a consequence of the various forms of social inequality and material disadvantage to which people can be subject throughout the course of their lives (Friedli 2009).

CHAPTER SUMMARY

This chapter has examined a variety of critical issues that are associated with how mental distress is understood, and, in particular, has reflected upon what contributes to the emergence and maintenance of that distress. In particular, it has critically considered the approach variously referred to as the biological, medical or biomedical model of mental distress, which has been, and continues to be, vigorously debated by those who work within and those who use mental health services. In contrast to that model's assumption that mental distress is a meaningless manifestation of some form of biological dysfunction or disease process, this chapter has also examined the emerging psychological and, in particular, trauma-informed approach to mental distress. In doing so, we have considered how such distress may be understood as a meaningful response to traumatic and adverse events that can occur at various stages of an individual's life and especially during a person's childhood. Finally, within the context of the enduring assumption that the origin of mental distress is primarily to be found within the individual – an assumption which has been associated with both biological and psychological approaches – this chapter has also examined the social determinants of mental distress. In doing so, we have discussed how a range of social, economic and political factors that are located outside or beyond the individual, and which can profoundly influence and determine the social and material conditions of an individual's life, have been implicated in the emergence and maintenance of mental distress.

ACTIVITIES: BRIEF OUTLINE ANSWERS

ACTIVITY 2.1 RESEARCH

In conducting your own research into Emil Kraepelin you may have discovered detailed information about who he was and what contribution he made to the development of a biological approach to mental distress. For example, you may have found out that Kraepelin was a late 19th-, early 20th-century German psychiatrist who is sometimes regarded as the 'father' of modern psychiatry. In part, this is because of his introduction of the influential diagnostic division between 'manic depression' and '*dementia praecox*' – the latter term being subsequently reformulated by the Swiss psychiatrist Eugen Bleuler as schizophrenia. It has also been suggested, however, that Kraepelin's importance is the result of his development of a new paradigm or way of thinking about mental distress (Bentall 2004).

Against the diagnostic confusion that characterised the period in which he developed his ideas, Kraepelin proposed that symptoms of mental distress which occurred together and appeared to follow a similar course were an indication of a particular type of 'psychiatric disorder'. In doing so, he assumed not only that there were a limited number of separate and naturally occurring psychiatric disorders that had their own set of symptoms or 'symptom profile', but also that each of those disorders would be found to correspond to a specific brain disease. In addition, he assumed that the identification of each separate psychiatric disorder in terms of its symptom profile, a profile which corresponded to a specific brain disease, would lead directly to an understanding of the cause of each of those psychiatric disorders.

ACTIVITY 2.2 TEAM WORKING

The reasons why the relationship between childhood trauma and adult mental distress is controversial, and why mental health professionals may be reluctant to recognise and respond to this relationship, is complex and contested. However, a variety of reasons have been proposed, many of which you may have discussed with your colleagues. For example, it has been suggested that practitioners have been reluctant to recognise and respond to trauma because of a lack of knowledge and skills to enable them to do so; for fear of offending, distressing or re-traumatising those who use mental health services; because of the enduring notion that mental distress has a primarily biological basis; and as a consequence of a belief that reports of childhood trauma expressed by those experiencing mental distress may be unreliable (Read *et al.* 2008; Herman 2015) – despite evidence to the contrary (Fisher *et al.* 2011).

It has also been suggested that there has been a reluctance to acknowledge the relationship between childhood trauma and adult mental distress because such a position has been understood as blaming and stigmatising families (Johnstone 2012). As a consequence, when family influence upon mental distress has been acknowledged it has been presented as a factor which may prevent recovery from pre-existing mental distress rather than contribute to its emergence (as with the notion of **high expressed emotion**). In addition, it has been claimed that there is a personal, professional and even societal tendency to deny and repress childhood trauma because of a reluctance to confront the reality of such events and the horrifying experiences that some people have been subjected to by others (Sweeney *et al.* 2016).

ACTIVITY 2.3 RESEARCH

In conducting your own research into Urie Bronfenbrenner's (1979) ecological systems theory you may have discovered that it was originally introduced as a theoretical perspective on childhood development. However, it has been used beyond that area to suggest that a person's health and happiness, as well as their difficulties and distress, can only be fully understood by recognising that each human being exists within, and is continuously influenced by, a number of interacting social systems. In particular, you may have found out that each person is understood as existing within an immediate social environment, or what is referred to as the microsystem, which can include a person's home life, their neighbourhood and their workplace. In contrast, the mesosystem is made up of the multiple interactions that exist within a person's microsystem, such as the reciprocal relationships that exist between a person's home life and their working environment.

You may also have discovered that a person's microsystem and mesosystem exist within a larger exosystem, which is composed of the settings, and the decisions taken in those settings, that exert an influence upon a person but in which they play no part. These can include local or national decisions on health and welfare expenditure or the availability of affordable housing. The exosystem belongs, in turn, to a larger socio-cultural environment, or what is referred to as the macrosystem, which is made up of a society's cultural values and norms, its political and economic systems as well as its relationships with other countries and their governments. Finally, the chronosystem adds the dimension of time to the preceding four social systems and highlights how changes in any one of those systems can have both direct and indirect consequences for a person's health and happiness as well as their difficulties and distress.

FURTHER READING

- **Bloom SL & Farragher B** (2013) *Restoring Sanctuary: A New Operating System for Trauma-Informed Systems of Care*. New York, NY: Oxford University Press.

This book examines how to facilitate individual and organisational change in a variety of care settings, and, by using the Sanctuary Model, how to create a safe, secure and trauma-informed approach to mental distress.

- **Compton MT & Shim RS** (eds) (2015) *Social Determinants of Mental Health*. Arlington, VA: American Psychiatric Publishing.

A comprehensive account of the social determinants of mental health that explores the implications of developing an awareness of these determinants for both clinical and policy decision-making in mental health care.

- **Cooke A** (ed) (2017) *Understanding Psychosis and Schizophrenia*. Leicester: The British Psychological Society.

This is an accessible and wide-ranging report that provides, among other things, a psychological account of those experiences that are associated with a diagnosis of schizophrenia and psychosis more generally.

- **Deacon B & McKay D** (2015) The biomedical model of psychological disorders. *the Behavior Therapist*, 38(7): 169–245.

A special issue of *the Behavior Therapist* which includes 11 stimulating articles providing critical analyses of different aspects of the biomedical model, written by notable figures working in various fields affiliated with mental health care.

- **Read J & Dillon J** (eds) (2013) *Models of Madness: Psychological, Social and Biological Approaches to Psychosis*, 2nd edition. Hove: Routledge.

An evidence-based critique of various aspects of the biological approach to mental distress that maintains the need for alternative psychological and sociological understandings and responses to that distress.

USEFUL WEBSITES

- www.intervoiceonline.org

This is the website for The International Hearing Voices Network, an organisation that aims to provide information, encourage research and promote an understanding of voice hearing as a potentially meaningful and empowering human experience.

- www.samhsa.gov/nctic

Here you will find the website for the National Center for Trauma-Informed Care that seeks to develop the knowledge base for, and facilitate the adoption of, trauma-informed approaches in the delivery of a broad range of human services.

3

PSYCHIATRIC DIAGNOSIS

CHAPTER AIMS

By the end of this chapter you will be able to:

- assess the legitimacy of psychiatric diagnoses;
- debate the value-laden character of psychiatric diagnoses;
- evaluate an alternative to the use of psychiatric diagnosis.

INTRODUCTION

CASE STUDY

Riya is in the second week of her clinical placement on an acute mental health unit and has just finished observing the weekly ward review. As she reflects upon the experience with her mentor William, she says that she has noticed how the difficulties experienced by service users/survivors, and the therapeutic responses to those difficulties, were discussed in the context of a variety of diagnoses. While she recognised some of the categories being used, such as schizophrenia and bipolar disorder, she tells William that she was unfamiliar with others, such as borderline personality disorder and schizoaffective disorder. William informs her that while there are many psychiatric diagnoses she should begin developing her knowledge of the characteristic symptoms of 'common' diagnoses used in the clinical area. In providing her with a list of these diagnoses he suggests that a knowledge of them will not only be important for understanding the various forms that mental distress can take but will also enable her to effectively communicate with other mental health professionals about that distress.

The use of psychiatric diagnosis is central to the discipline of psychiatry and contemporary mental health care. As noted by Riya in the above case study, the experiences of those who use mental health services are commonly understood in the context of diagnostic categories and the symptoms that are associated with those categories. In this way, psychiatric diagnoses not only provide an established framework for organising and comprehending the sometimes complex, unusual and disturbing experiences that can be associated with mental distress; rather, in so far as they provide a vocabulary that is understood and shared by many, psychiatric diagnoses also enable mental health professionals to coherently communicate their clinical understandings with others and to consider, negotiate and determine interventions on the basis of those shared understandings. However, despite its centrality in contemporary mental health care, psychiatric diagnosis has been, and continues to be, subject to sustained critique (Frances 2013; Pilgrim 2014; Timimi 2014). For example, there are critical discussions about the conceptual status of psychiatric diagnoses and the extent to which they accurately identify supposedly distinct and naturally occurring disorders. There are also ongoing concerns about the role that social, cultural and historical values and norms have in psychiatric diagnostic systems and the effect of those values and norms upon the diagnostic judgements of mental health professionals. In addition, there are political and philosophical analyses of the proliferation of psychiatric diagnoses in contemporary mental health care and throughout society, as well as critical considerations about the consequences of those diagnoses for the lives of those who receive them.

The purpose of this chapter is therefore to introduce you to a variety of critical issues surrounding the theoretical basis and the clinical employment of psychiatric diagnosis in contemporary mental health care. It will begin by critically considering the legitimacy of existing diagnostic categories and the extent to which they accurately identify, and draw clear boundaries between, supposedly distinct and naturally occurring biologically based mental disorders. In contrast to the notion that psychiatric diagnosis is a scientific, objective and value-free enterprise, we shall then examine the manner in which various social, cultural and historical values are implicated in the use of diagnostic categories. In particular, this chapter will propose that a recognition of how psychiatric diagnosis is made 'against a background' of such values and norms challenges the way in which that practice seeks to legitimise itself as being concerned with the identification of naturally occurring biologically based disorders. Finally, we shall conclude by considering an alternative to psychiatric diagnosis that has been most closely associated with the discipline of clinical psychology and is commonly referred to as 'psychological formulation' or simply 'formulation'. Understanding this as a contrasting approach to psychiatric diagnosis, this chapter will examine how the thoughts, feelings and behaviours that are associated with mental distress can be recognised as meaningful once they are considered, through the use of formulation, in the unique context of a person's life history and current circumstances.

THE LEGITIMACY OF PSYCHIATRIC DIAGNOSIS

ACTIVITY 3.1 RESEARCH

In 1973 the American psychologist David Rosenhan published the results of one of the most famous research experiments in the history of psychiatry in the prestigious journal *Science*. Among other things, the experiment powerfully illustrated a variety of critical issues surrounding the legitimacy of psychiatric diagnosis and the ability of mental health professionals to distinguish everyday human behaviour from mental distress.

For this activity conduct your own research into Rosenhan's study, entitled 'On being sane in insane places', and provide a brief overview of its aims, methods and results. In doing so, attempt to summarise the conclusions that Rosenhan draws from the study and the ability of mental health professionals to use the notions of 'normality and abnormality, sanity and insanity, and the diagnoses that flow from them' (Rosenhan 1973, p. 250).

An outline answer is provided at the end of the chapter.

To begin to understand the critical issues surrounding the legitimacy of psychiatric diagnosis, it is productive to consider the manner in which that practice is said to have gained its legitimacy in contemporary mental health care and throughout Western societies. In particular, it has been suggested that psychiatric diagnosis has gained that legitimacy by presenting itself as being equivalent to medical diagnosis and as being a practice that is therefore concerned with the reliable and valid categorisation of supposedly distinct and naturally occurring biologically based medical disorders (Moncrieff 2010; Boyle 2012). Indeed, contemporary psychiatric classification is said to reflect a specific paradigm, framework or way of thinking about mental distress (the articulation of which is attributed to the late 19th-century German psychiatrist Emil Kraepelin) that is comprised of a number of assumptions that are drawn from other branches of medicine and from the natural sciences in general (Pilgrim 2014; Hoff 2015). This Kraepelinian – or, more precisely, neo-Kraepelinian framework – suggests that, firstly, there exist distinct and naturally occurring 'mental disorders' which are characterised by their own specific set of symptoms; secondly, there are not only clear boundaries between those separate disorders, but there is a clear division between 'mental health' and 'mental illness'; and thirdly, the variety of separate mental disorders, in accordance with the biological approach to mental distress, are a consequence of various forms of neurobiological deficit or dysfunction (Klerman 1978; Bentall 2010).

Despite seeking to present itself as being engaged in the same diagnostic practice as other branches of medicine, the supposed equivalence of psychiatric diagnosis with medical diagnosis has been a matter of ongoing debate. For example, it has been suggested that psychiatric diagnosis differs significantly from diagnosis in other areas and, while a variety of differences have been proposed, one of the most fundamental is concerned with the detection and assessment of **signs** and **symptoms**. The practice of diagnosis in any area of health care is a complex process in which variability exists in how health care professionals arrive at a diagnosis. However, it has been suggested that in order to do so in a reliable and valid way both signs and symptoms are necessary (Boyle 2012). Symptoms are understood as referring to the bodily complaints, personal accounts and subjective experiences that people commonly report to practitioners, such as dizziness, blurred vision or stomach ache. In contrast, signs are the far less ambiguous physical indicators of the potential presence of a disease or disorder, such as a low white blood cell count, an irregular pulse rate or high blood pressure. Although symptoms can provide the first indication of potential health care problems, they can be highly subjective and can have many possible causes. Therefore, rather than relying on symptoms alone, the presence of a disease or disorder in medicine is confirmed when those symptoms are associated with signs and the physical manifestation of a disease that can be detected by a variety of medical measures such as blood tests, x-rays and tissue samples.

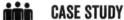 **CASE STUDY**

Kelvin is a 19-year-old university student who was admitted to an acute mental health unit eight weeks ago and has since received a diagnosis of schizophrenia. Although his older brother Godwin lives abroad, he has travelled to visit Kelvin and is currently talking to Lara, a mental health professional on the ward, about why his brother has received that diagnosis. Lara explains that, prior to his admission, Kelvin's university lecturers reported that his academic work had significantly deteriorated over a period of six months, while his friends had noticed that he was expressing 'odd beliefs' and behaviour that was 'out of character'. Moreover, Lara tells Godwin that, following admission, Kelvin has been observed to display a variety of symptoms that are associated with a diagnosis of schizophrenia. In particular, she says that Kelvin has been expressing 'bizarre delusional beliefs' and his speech is often 'disorganised', switching rapidly from one topic to another. In addition, Lara informs Godwin that Kelvin's behaviour is also 'disorganised' and has been characterised by a significant degree of 'excitement', 'restlessness' and 'unpredictable agitation'.

In contrast to the diagnosis of disorders in other areas of medicine, for the majority of cases there are no signs by which the identification of supposedly distinct biologically based mental disorders can be made. As was discussed in the previous chapter, it has been suggested that there is a lack of reliable, replicable and therefore compelling evidence for a clear biological cause in many forms of mental distress (Cromby *et al.* 2013; Deacon 2013). Therefore, despite ongoing research into their existence, there are no physiological indicators or **biomarkers** that can be used to confirm the presence of particular forms of mental distress (Scarr *et al.* 2015;

Venkatasubramanian & Keshavan 2016). As a consequence, there are no signs that can be detected by medical measures to confirm a psychiatric diagnosis, which is to say that there exist no blood tests, x-rays or tissue samples to confirm a diagnosis of, for example, schizophrenia, bipolar disorder or depression. Rather, as in the above case study, a psychiatric diagnosis is made exclusively on the basis of symptoms, without the ability to associate those symptoms with signs and the physical manifestation of an underlying biological disorder. In particular, the diagnostic judgements of mental health professionals are based exclusively on a consideration of a person's feelings, thoughts and behaviour, the accounts of which are either offered by the person experiencing mental distress or by others (such as friends, relatives or neighbours) who have some form of association with that person.

CONCEPT SUMMARY: THE DIAGNOSTIC AND STATISTICAL MANUAL

Produced by the American Psychiatric Association, the *Diagnostic and Statistical Manual of Mental Disorders* (DSM) provides a comprehensive description of the various diagnostic categories that can be used to classify a person's experience of mental distress. In doing so, the DSM presents a precise list of symptoms for each psychiatric diagnosis along with specific rules that state, for example, how many symptoms are required for a diagnosis to be made and the length of time that the symptoms must have been present. While the DSM was first published in 1952, it is periodically subject to revision and new editions are published following a process of consultation. During this process the legitimacy of existing diagnoses is discussed and new diagnostic categories are proposed by panels of health care professionals before being approved for inclusion in the latest edition of the DSM by a central committee of American Psychiatric Association members.

In Europe and the United Kingdom the official diagnostic system is the *International Classification of Diseases* (ICD), which is published by the World Health Organization and undergoes similar periodic revisions as the DSM. Of the two diagnostic systems the DSM is internationally the most influential and its categories are recognised around the world for both clinical and research purposes. While minor differences exist between the two systems, both maintain the neo-Kraepelinian assumption that mental distress can be divided into distinct biologically based disorders. For example, while acknowledging 'a complete description of the underlying pathological processes that is not possible for most mental disorders' (APA 2013, p.xli), and that 'the boundaries between disorders are more porous than originally perceived' (APA 2013, p. 6), the fifth and most recent edition of the DSM proposes that it 'remains a categorical classification of separate disorders' and 'the best available description of how mental disorders are expressed' (APA 2013, p. xli).

That psychiatric diagnosis is made exclusively on the basis of symptoms without recourse to signs can be understood as presenting a considerable challenge to the legitimacy of psychiatric diagnosis. Without the ability to associate psychiatric symptoms with signs, or the ability to link the personal accounts of mental distress with some form of underlying disease process, there is no clear indication that those symptoms or experiences are an expression of a distinct biologically based disorder.

In illustrating this challenge to the legitimacy of psychiatric diagnosis, it has been suggested that – rather than being equivalent to the practice of medical diagnosis – mental health professionals are in a position that is somewhat similar to a medical doctor, who, for some reason, has no access to standard medical measures such as blood tests, x-rays and tissue samples (Johnstone 2008). Despite not having these measures, the doctor proceeds to give a person a diagnosis of diabetes on the basis of a variety of reported symptoms, including that person's account of feeling tired, having blurred vision and of experiencing weight loss. However, the doctor has no way to associate those symptoms with signs, no medical measures by which to link the person's reported symptoms with an underlying disease process and therefore no conclusive way of deciding whether that person's tiredness, blurred vision and weight loss are a result of diabetes rather than, for example, cancer, poor nutrition or simply the chance coexistence of a number of separate complaints.

─────── PRACTICE ISSUE: RELIABILITY AND VALIDITY ───────

The notions of reliability and validity have specific, technical meanings in the context of discussions about the legitimacy of psychiatric diagnosis. Reliability refers to the consistency with which diagnostic categories are used and is assessed by investigating the extent to which two or more practitioners agree about the diagnosis a person has been given, or the consistency with which one practitioner uses a particular diagnosis on two different occasions. Although the reliability of psychiatric diagnosis has historically been poor there has been a continued focus upon the attempt to improve the consistency with which diagnostic categories are used in mental health care. For example, the attempt to address the problem of reliability was a significant motivating factor in the production of the third and most influential edition of the *Diagnostic and Statistical Manual* (Lieberman 2016). However, while the reliability of psychiatric diagnosis is said to have improved (particularly in those research settings in which structured diagnostic interviews are used) it has been argued that in routine clinical practice (in which diagnostic categories are used in a less structured manner) the reliability of psychiatric diagnosis remains limited (Bentall 2010; Whooley 2010; Newnes 2014).

In contrast to reliability, validity is a philosophically complex notion that is commonly understood as referring to how a given category, to use Plato's memorable phrase, 'carves nature at its joints' (*Phaedrus* 265e). That is, validity designates the degree to which a diagnostic category meaningfully represents a specific feature of the world and, rather than being an artificial distinction, accurately identifies or 'picks out' a separate and naturally occurring disorder (Hempel 1994). While the focus has been upon improving the reliability of psychiatric diagnoses, it is important to recognise that even if complete reliability could be achieved this would not establish the validity of those diagnoses. For example, throughout the history of psychiatry there have been a variety of diagnoses (most notoriously **hysteria**, homosexuality and **drapetomania**) that have been formulated in such a way as to enable different practitioners to agree who should receive those diagnoses and to thereby use them in a consistent and reliable manner, but which, despite this reliability, are no longer understood as identifying mental disorders and are therefore no longer considered to be valid psychiatric diagnoses (Scull 2011; Greenberg 2013).

Although psychiatric diagnosis is said to have gained its legitimacy by presenting itself as being equivalent to medical diagnosis, without the ability to link psychiatric symptoms with signs (and with some form of underlying biological dysfunction in particular) there is no conclusive way of deciding whether existing psychiatric diagnoses accurately identify, and draw clear boundaries between, supposedly separate forms of mental distress. Indeed, symptoms that supposedly characterise one psychiatric diagnosis may be experienced by people who have been given an alternative diagnosis, and this coexistence or overlap of symptoms has contributed to an increased awareness that the boundaries between different diagnoses may be less distinct than previously thought. For example, the recognition that a significant number of people have experiences that are associated with a diagnosis of both schizophrenia and bipolar disorder has contributed to claims that the traditional division between the two (a division which has its origins in Emil Kraepelin's distinction between *dementia praecox* and manic depression) does not reflect a naturally occurring division between two separate forms of mental distress (Lake 2012; Pearlson 2015). Rather, it has been suggested that the 'psychotic and affective experiences' that are associated with schizophrenia and bipolar disorder exist along a continuum (Crow 2010; Keshavan *et al.* 2011), such that those two separate diagnostic categories should therefore be replaced with a single term, such as 'psychosis spectrum syndrome', to reflect this continuity (van Os 2016).

In addition to critical concerns about whether existing psychiatric diagnoses meaningfully represent, and accurately draw clear boundaries between, supposedly distinct forms of mental distress, the neo-Kraepelinian assumption that there exists a clear division between 'mental health' and 'mental illness' has also been disputed. In part, this has emerged as a result of research which indicates that those 'psychotic experiences' which are associated with schizophrenia – such as hearing voices and unusual beliefs – are found among the general population and for many people are not associated with a discernible impairment in everyday functioning or the need for mental health care (Beaven *et al.* 2011; Linscott & van Os 2013). Such research has been used to support the suggestion that, rather than necessarily being an indication of a mental disorder, psychotic experiences may exist upon a continuum consistent with 'normal experience' (DeRosse & Karlsgodt 2015; Rössler *et al.* 2015). In particular, the prevalence of voice hearing and unusual beliefs in the general population has led to claims that such experiences may be more productively understood as a normal human variation. Moreover, it has been suggested that the way in which these experiences can contribute to mental distress is not simply a result of the character of those experiences, such as their intensity, frequency and persistence; rather, it is also influenced by a person's assessment of, and response to, those experiences, along with the social, cultural and historical context in which such experiences occur (Romme & Escher 1989; Peters *et al.* 2012).

VALUES, NORMS AND PSYCHIATRIC DIAGNOSIS

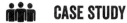 **CASE STUDY**

Now in her late twenties, Khanyi became involved with mental health services while still a teenager. Following repeated instances of self-harm and reports of 'challenging', 'disruptive' and 'inappropriate' behaviour, she was initially given a number of provisional diagnoses. Several years ago, however, she was given a diagnosis of borderline personality disorder (although she questions, disputes and sometimes explicitly rejects that diagnosis). Although Khanyi has not been admitted to hospital in a while she repeatedly presents to mental health services in a state of distress at varying times of the night and day. In doing so, she often displays outbursts of anger and aggression and suggests that people 'always let her down'; on other occasions she reports having feelings of intense sadness and guilt, believing that she is fundamentally 'weak', 'bad' or 'evil'. She sometimes maintains that she is 'powerless' or 'hollow inside' and periodically suggests that she feels as though she 'doesn't really exist'. Moreover, since the beginning of her involvement with mental health services she has continued to engage in self-harm behaviours and often lacerates her forearms, which, on occasion, require medical intervention.

Arguably the most enduring critical debates surrounding the use of psychiatric diagnoses are concerned with the way in which social, cultural and historical values and norms are thought to be implicated in the diagnostic categories employed in psychiatry and the diagnostic judgements of mental health professionals (Thornton 2007). In order to begin to understand these critical debates, it is productive to recognise that while psychiatric diagnosis is made on the basis of symptoms without recourse to signs (and without the ability to associate those symptoms with some form of biological dysfunction), the content of those symptoms is not, in contrast with other branches of medicine, typically characterised by a person's concerns about some aspect of their body. That is, the symptoms that mental health professionals take into consideration when developing their diagnostic judgements are not commonly concerned with a person's subjective experience of some form of disturbance in their physiological functioning such as dizziness, blurred vision or stomach ache. Rather, the judgement that a person is experiencing a particular form of mental distress and should therefore receive a specific psychiatric diagnosis is made following a consideration of that person's feelings, thoughts and behaviour – such as those displayed by Khanyi in the above case study – the accounts of which are either offered by the person experiencing such distress or by others who have some form of association with that person.

It has been suggested, however, that in order to make diagnostic judgements in mental health care, and to base those judgements on a person's feelings, thoughts and behaviour, then it is necessary to do so in the context or 'against the background' of what are considered to be 'ordered' or 'normal' feelings, thoughts and behaviour (Szasz 1960; Stier 2013). However, while it is said to be possible to establish what is the ordered or normal functioning of the human body in a relatively uncontroversial way (to reach a consensus, for example, about what the normal range of blood pressure ought to be), the ability to establish what are ordered or normal feelings, thoughts and behaviour is substantially more controversial. In particular, the notion of normal thoughts, feelings and behaviour (notions which can serve as the background against which a psychiatric diagnosis can be made) is dependent upon a range of often unarticulated and even unacknowledged value judgements or **normative assumptions** about how people ought to think, feel and behave. Indeed, it has been suggested that all systems of psychiatric classification, and the diagnostic categories which belong to them, are not only influenced by the interests and needs of those who develop such systems, but they also reflect the values and norms of the particular societies, cultures and historical periods in which they are developed (Bentall 2010; Busfield 2014).

CONCEPT SUMMARY: THE 'DISORDERED' PERSONALITY

Among the range of psychiatric diagnoses that are used in contemporary mental health care, personality disorders are arguably the most controversial. While a variety of critical issues surround these diagnostic categories, one of the most fundamental is concerned with how the criteria that are used to make those diagnoses reflect a variety of social, cultural and historical value judgements about how people ought to think, feel and behave. For example, the *Diagnostic and Statistical Manual* presents 'Cluster B Personality Disorders' (which includes antisocial, borderline, narcissistic and histrionic personality disorders) as being variously characterised by 'deceitfulness', 'irresponsibility', 'unstable relationships', 'inappropriate anger', 'grandiosity' and 'arrogant, haughty behaviours', as well as 'excessive emotionality' and 'inappropriate sexually seductive or provocative behaviour' (APA 2013, pp. 659–672).

It has been suggested, however, that such criteria require mental health professionals to employ a variety of normative assumptions and make a range of value judgements in order to decide, for example, what constitutes an excessive versus a proportionate expression of emotion. In addition, it has also been argued that the thoughts, feelings and behaviours which supposedly characterise a 'disordered' personality imply a social, cultural and historical conception of an 'ordered' or an 'undisordered' personality – a personality which is, for example, characterised by honesty, emotional stability and sexual modesty. Consequently, it has been suggested that this conception of an ordered personality has served as the moral, rather than the medical, background against which the notion of personality disorder and its associated diagnostic categories have been developed (Charland 2006; Leising *et al.* 2009).

In presenting itself as being equivalent to medical diagnosis, and as being a practice that is concerned with the reliable and valid categorisation of biologically based medical disorders, psychiatric diagnosis has sought to legitimise itself as an endeavour that is scientific, objective and free of value judgements. Moreover, it has been suggested that the presence of values and norms in any aspect of psychiatric diagnosis introduces an unacceptable degree of 'subjective bias' into that practice, such that there should be an attempt to remove all values and norms from psychiatry's diagnostic judgements, categories and systems (Hempel 1994; Sisti *et al.* 2013). However, rather than being unique to psychiatric diagnosis, it has been suggested that values and norms are implicated in the notions of health, illness and disease in any branch of medicine, in so far as these notions reflect a variety of human concerns and value judgements about which physiological states are desirable and which are not (King 1954). Indeed, in highlighting the variety of 'natural events' with which medicine is concerned – including 'fractures of bones, the fatal ruptures of tissues, the malignant multiplication of tumorous growths' – Sedgwick (1982) has proposed that 'these, as natural events, do not constitute illnesses, sicknesses or diseases prior to the social meanings we attach to them' such that, prior to this attachment of meaning, '*there are no illnesses or diseases in nature*' (p. 30).

While they are often unarticulated and unacknowledged, the presence of value judgements in any area of health care – and within the diagnostic judgements and categories which characterise those areas – is therefore said to be ineliminable (Stier 2013). Accordingly, rather than seeking to somehow remove all values and norms from the practice of psychiatric diagnosis, it is necessary to acknowledge the manner in which they can be a feature of that practice. In particular, it has been suggested that it is necessary to consider critically how value judgements can affect the theory and practice of mental health care in both productive and non-productive ways, and to do so with the collaborative participation of mental health professionals, those who use mental health services and the wider public (Fulford *et al.* 2005; Sisti *et al.* 2013). Moreover, rather than necessarily being undermined by the presence of values, a central critical concern about psychiatric diagnosis is the manner in which it has presented itself as a value-free practice that identifies biologically based medical disorders when such diagnoses are made against a background of social, cultural and historical value judgements. For example, while maintaining that values and norms are necessarily implicated in the identification of mental distress, and that there is nothing intrinsically wrong with this state of affairs, Johnstone (2013) has made it clear that 'the problem arises when subjectivity is presented as objectivity, or to put it another way, when social and cultural judgements are presented as if they were medical ones about bodily problems' (p. 109).

——————— CONCEPT SUMMARY: PSYCHIATRIC IMPERIALISM ———————

By seeking to legitimise itself as being concerned with the detection of biologically based medical disorders, psychiatric diagnosis is said to have given insufficient attention to how its categories reflect a range of value judgements, normative assumptions and philosophical presuppositions that are characteristic of the West (Summerfield 2012). In its 'Glossary of Cultural Concepts of Distress', for example, the *Diagnostic and Statistical Manual* provides an overview of how other cultures understand and respond to mental distress in alternative ways. However, it has been argued that by placing this overview in the Appendix, the impression is created that the preceding diagnostic categories (such as schizophrenia, depression and personality disor-der) are universal or transcultural categories that can be applied across all cultures rather than reflecting Western cultural concepts of distress (Watters 2011).

In the context of the increasing dominance of Western medicine around the world, and the **movement for global mental health** in particular (Patel *et al.* 2011), the idea of Western psychiatric diagnoses as value-free and applicable across all cultures has meant that minimal consideration has been given to how those cultures understand and respond to mental distress. Indeed, the dominance and spread of Western psychiatric diagnoses around the world is said to be responsible for a marginalisation, depreciation and even elimination of different cultural understandings of distress. Analogous to the West's historical colonisation of non-Western cul-tures, this process has been presented as an 'imperialism' of Western ideas about mental distress and an unremitting expansion of the value judgements, normative assumptions and philosophical presuppositions that are associated with those ideas (Fernando 2010; Mills 2014).

To maintain that values and norms are a feature of the diagnostic categories employed in psychiatry and the diagnostic judgements of mental health profession-als is not to suggest that the experiences which can be associated with mental distress should somehow be understood as 'less credible' or 'less real' than the dis-tress which characterises other areas of health care. As you will almost certainly be aware, the experiences of those who use mental health services can be intense, alarming and even profoundly disturbing, both for the person experiencing mental distress and for those who have an association with that person. Therefore, rather than invalidating the experiences associated with mental distress, a recognition of how psychiatric diagnosis is made against a background of values and norms calls into question the idea of diagnosis as a value-free practice and requires a critical consideration of the implications of perpetuating this idea. For example, it has been suggested that understanding psychiatric diagnosis as a value-free endeavour that is concerned with the categorisation of biologically based medical disorders can restrict an understanding of how other non-biological factors can contribute to mental distress (Boyle 2011). In particular, the notion that psychiatric diagnosis is equivalent to medical diagnosis can obscure how the experiences that are associated with mental distress may be more productively understood as meaningful responses to a range of adverse life events and challenging circumstances to which people can be subject during the course of their lives.

--------- **PRACTICE ISSUE: THE MYTH OF MENTAL ILLNESS** ---------

At the beginning of his influential paper, 'The myth of mental illness', Thomas Szasz (1983) makes the following startling assertion: 'My aim in this essay is to ask if there is such a thing as mental illness, and to argue that there is not' (p. 12). In doing so, however, he does not suggest that the various experiences which can be associated with mental distress do not

(Continued)

exist or are less real than the distress which characterises other areas of health care. As he makes clear, 'While I maintain that mental illnesses do not exist, I obviously do not imply or mean that the social and psychological occurrences to which this label is attached also do not exist' (Szasz 1983, p. 21). Rather, he argues that the various manifestations of distress that have traditionally been referred to as 'mental illnesses' are more productively understood as 'problems in living'.

Such problems in living arise as a consequence of the 'stress, strain and disharmony' that can characterise human relations as well as the contemporary challenge of attempting to give purpose and meaning to one's life (Szasz 1983, pp. 20–22). However, to refer to these problems in living as mental 'illnesses' – and to attach a variety of psychiatric diagnoses to the personal, social and existential problems that people can experience – is to conceal their real character. Szasz therefore maintains that the attempt to present these problems as biologically based medical disorders is inappropriate. In particular, he argues that the notion of mental illness is a 'disguise', a 'social tranquillizer' or a 'myth' that serves to obscure the personal, social and existential character of the problems in living that many people confront and are struggling to address (1983, pp. 21–23).

ACTIVITY 3.2   REFLECTION

Rather than being understood as the symptoms of a biologically based medical disorder, it has been suggested that the thoughts, feelings and behaviours that are associated with a diagnosis of borderline personality disorder can be more productively understood as meaningful responses to, and strategies for coping with, adverse life events and a range of challenging circumstances (Gunn & Potter 2015).

For this activity reflect critically on Khanyi's thoughts, feelings and behaviours as presented in the above case study. As you do so, consider how they might be better understood as meaningful responses to, and strategies for coping with, adverse life events and challenging circumstances rather than as the symptoms of a biologically based mental disorder.

An outline answer is provided at the end of the chapter.

PSYCHOLOGICAL FORMULATION

The use of psychiatric diagnosis, as was highlighted at the beginning of this chapter, is central to contemporary mental health care, and a variety of professional interests have been implicated in its continued use. For example, in seeking to present itself as being equivalent to medical diagnosis it has been suggested that psychiatric diagnosis is fundamental to psychiatry's ongoing concern to establish itself as a legitimate branch of medicine (Bentall 2010). It is important to recognise, however, that the continued use of psychiatric diagnosis can not only be understood as serving the interests of psychiatry and the concerns of the agencies, organisations and institutions with which that discipline is associated; rather, while those who receive a psychiatric diagnosis express a diverse range of opinions about the experience and its effects, the continued use of psychiatric diagnosis has been presented as potentially having various productive consequences for those who use mental health services. For example, the provision of certain forms of financial assistance, access to mental health services and a range of therapeutic interventions can be dependent upon receiving a psychiatric diagnosis. Moreover, in so far as it is associated with a biomedical explanation for the sometimes complex, confusing and disturbing experiences that can be associated with mental distress, it has been suggested that receiving a psychiatric diagnosis can provide a person with an accessible explanation for those experiences and this can contribute to a sense of comfort, relief and reassurance about their occurrence (Pitt *et al.* 2009).

Despite serving a variety of professional interests, psychiatric diagnosis can have a range of unproductive consequences that can potentially restrict and even prevent the attempt to facilitate therapeutic and recovery-orientated approaches in mental health care. For example, psychiatric diagnoses are associated with a variety of negative stereotypical assumptions, including the beliefs that people who receive such diagnoses are weak, unpredictable or dangerous. As a consequence, a person may not only be subject to various forms of stigma and **discrimination** on the basis of those diagnoses, but they can also come to understand themselves in accordance with such beliefs and this can contribute to a personal sense of hopelessness, helplessness and isolation (Ben-Zeev *et al.* 2010). Moreover, by being associated with an understanding of mental distress as a biologically based medical disorder, a psychiatric diagnosis can contribute to the positioning of a person in what has been referred to as the **sick role** (Johnstone 2000). Rather than being active participants in their own recovery, such an understanding of mental distress can lead a person to give responsibility for addressing that distress to medical professionals and to accept passively whatever treatment is recommended. Finally, in so far as a person who receives a psychiatric diagnosis comes to understand their mental distress in biomedical terms, then their own understanding of what may have contributed to that distress can become marginalised (Honos-Webb & Leitner 2001). Understood as a manifestation of some form of biological dysfunction, the need for mental health professionals to understand a person's mental distress in the unique context of their life history and current circumstances, and to collaboratively explore the meaning of such distress for that person, can come to be seen as unnecessary, unproductive and even irrelevant.

👥 CASE STUDY

After his mother remarried when he was six years old, Dylan's childhood changed dramatically. He suggests that his stepfather was 'violent and abusive' towards him over a four-year period and he was repeatedly told that the abuse occurred because of his own 'bad behaviour'. At the age of 10 Dylan's stepfather died suddenly, and shortly afterwards he attempted to tell his

(Continued)

mother about the abuse to which he had been subjected. However, Dylan's mother dismissed his account as 'nonsense' and he recalls that he subsequently made the decision to keep his difficulties to himself and 'never trust others'. In spite of his childhood, he did well at school and was the first person in his family to go to university. While there Dylan made a small number of friends and although he lost contact with his mother he remained in contact with his older sister Mary with whom he says he continues to have a good relationship.

Shortly after graduating from university, Dylan was offered what he described as his 'dream job' at a prestigious marketing company. Despite being located a long distance away from his sister and his university friends, he readily accepted the post. However, although he worked hard to try and impress his new employer, he found the competitive atmosphere of his work environment challenging and regularly began to work into the early hours of the morning. While he had not contacted Mary for over three months, she reports receiving a phone call at two o'clock yesterday morning from Dylan, who, in a very agitated state, told her that he had just had a serious argument with his colleagues. In particular, he told Mary that all of his colleagues were 'out to get him' and, although she found it difficult to fully make sense of what he was saying, that they were using 'some kind of device' to monitor, disrupt and steal his ideas.

The variety of critical concerns about the legitimacy of psychiatric diagnosis, and its potentially negative consequences for those who use mental health services, has contributed to the development of various initiatives that seek to provide alternatives to its use. While we shall discuss in Chapter 6 how some service users/ survivors have sought to resist psychiatric diagnosis, and thereby 'reclaim' their experience, we shall here consider an alternative that has been most closely associated with the discipline of clinical psychology and that is commonly referred to as 'psychological formulation' or simply 'formulation'. Although formulation has been defined in a variety of ways, in its broadest sense it can be understood as a hypothesis, plausible account or 'best guess' about what might have contributed to the emergence and the maintenance of a person's mental distress, and, on the basis of that account, what interventions might be helpful (Corrie & Lane 2010; Johnstone & Dallos 2014). Importantly, a formulation not only draws upon psychological theory and research into the manner in which a variety of adverse life events and wider social determinants can contribute to mental distress; rather, the development of a formulation is further situated within the unique context of a person's life and places central importance on a collaborative exploration of that person's understanding of the factors that may have contributed to their experience of mental distress, as well as the personal meaning that the experience may have for that individual.

In contrast to psychiatric diagnosis, therefore, a formulation does not understand mental distress as a consequence of some form of biological dysfunction that possesses no additional meaning beyond such biological processes. Rather, the fundamental assumption that guides the development of a formulation is that the thoughts, feelings and behaviours that are associated with mental distress, no matter how complex, unusual or disturbing they are, can on some level be understood as making sense once they are considered in the unique context of a person's life history and current circumstances (Butler 1998). It is important to recognise, however, that in seeking to make sense of what might have contributed to, and what might be perpetuating, a person's experience of mental distress, formulation can be an ongoing process rather than a single event. As new information and new understandings emerge during the collaborative development of a formulation, it will need to be revised to reflect those changes. Thus, formulation is not to be understood as somehow uncovering the 'real' or definitive account of what has caused a person's experience of mental distress, but is instead a provisional and dynamic account that is always open to reformulation and further refinement. Indeed, rather than being judged in terms of its truthfulness, it has been suggested that a formulation should be considered in terms of its usefulness and the extent to which it provides a productive understanding of a person's experience of mental distress that incorporates the meaning they give to that experience (Butler 1998).

CONCEPT SUMMARY: THE FOUR FACTORS MODEL

As with any clinical intervention, the ability to devise a useful formulation can take time to develop and will need to be practised regularly. To facilitate this process the four factors model suggests that a productive way to guide the development of a formulation is to consider four factors that may have contributed to, and may be maintaining, a person's experience of mental distress (Read & Sanders 2011).

- **Predisposing** factors are those events that have occurred early in a person's life and which increase the possibility of developing mental distress later in life. They can be external events such as trauma and adverse social circumstances, or they can be internal attributes such as having low self-esteem or being suspicious of others.
- **Precipitating** factors are those occurrences which can incite or trigger a person's experience of mental distress, sometimes by interacting with their predisposing factors. For example, a person who developed low self-esteem in childhood may become anxious or depressed when they experience a perceived failure in adulthood.
- **Perpetuating** factors are those ongoing occurrences which can maintain a person's experience of mental distress. Again, these can be external events such as poor housing, insecure employment or isolation, or they can be internal attributes such as the belief that you are worthless or that asking for assistance is a sign of weakness.
- **Preventative** factors are those things that a person has or does to alleviate or to protect themselves from the emergence and maintenance of mental distress. These can be personal strengths and capabilities or external things in which a person participates, such as recreational activities or social support groups.

Despite recognising its value in understanding a person's experience of mental distress, formulation is commonly understood by mental health professionals as something that can be used alongside, rather than being an alternative to, psychiatric diagnosis (Mohtashemi *et al.* 2016). However, it has been argued that psychiatric diagnosis and formulation are based upon such radically different theoretical assumptions that they cannot be understood as complementary approaches to understanding a person's experience of mental distress. As we have suggested, a psychiatric diagnosis is associated with an understanding of mental distress as a biologically based medical disorder that has no additional meaning beyond such biological disorder. Moreover, in so far as psychiatric diagnoses are based upon the judgements of mental health professionals, the person's understanding of what might have contributed to their mental distress can become marginalised. In contrast, the fundamental assumption of formulation is that a person's experience of mental distress makes sense and, through a collaborative exploration with the person about what might have led to its emergence, can be understood in the unique context of their life. Indeed, once a formulation has been developed to explain a person's experiences or 'complaints' – such as low mood, hearing voices or unusual beliefs – then it has been suggested that the use of a psychiatric diagnosis becomes unnecessary and adds nothing meaningful to an understanding of what has contributed to those complaints. As Bentall (2010) makes clear, 'Once the complaints have been explained, there will be no "schizophrenia" and "bipolar disorder" left behind to explain afterwards' (p. 166).

ACTIVITY 3.3   TEAM WORKING

While formulations are commonly developed within the context of individual therapeutic encounters, there is increasing interest in the development of formulations within the context of teams (Cole *et al.* 2015). In team formulation a number of mental health professionals from a variety of disciplinary backgrounds share their skills, knowledge and experience in order to develop an account of a person's experience of mental distress, and, on the basis of that account, determine what interventions might be helpful.

For this activity consider Dylan's mental distress in the case study above. With your colleagues attempt to develop a provisional team formulation about what may have contributed to that distress and, in particular, his unusual beliefs about his co-workers. In order to structure the development of your team formulation use the four factors model outlined above and, as you do so, resist explaining Dylan's thoughts, feelings and behaviour by referring to psychiatric categories and diagnoses.

An outline answer is provided at the end of the chapter.

It is important to recognise that formulation is not without its limitations and a variety of critical concerns about its use as an alternative to psychiatric diagnosis have been identified. For example, it has been suggested that the development of a formulation can be time consuming, and, within the context of the enduring influence of biological approaches to mental distress, there can be a pressure on practitioners to provide a psychiatric diagnosis – a pressure which may not only come from other health care professionals but also from those who use mental health services (Mohtashemi *et al.* 2016). In addition, while formulation emphasises the importance of working collaboratively with those who experience mental distress, there are concerns about the extent to which practitioners are able to accommodate a person's understanding of mental distress when it challenges the social, cultural and historical assumptions of the psychological theories used to develop a formulation. Moreover, in the context of evidence-based practice in contemporary mental health care, it has been suggested that more research is required into various aspects of the use of formulation (Johnstone & Dallos 2014). For example, there is a need to investigate further how formulation is implemented in the clinical area, the manner in which it enables an effective therapeutic response to mental distress and the extent to which those who use mental health services value formulation as a process that provides a more productive understanding of such distress in comparison with that provided by psychiatric diagnosis.

CHAPTER SUMMARY

This chapter has introduced a variety of critical issues surrounding the theoretical basis and the clinical employment of psychiatric diagnosis in contemporary mental health care. In doing so, it has critically considered the legitimacy of existing diagnostic categories and the extent to which they accurately identify, and draw clear boundaries between, supposedly distinct and naturally occurring biologically based mental disorders. Moreover, in contrast to the presentation of psychiatric diagnosis as a scientific, objective and value-free enterprise, we have examined the manner in which a variety of social, cultural and historical values and norms are implicated in the use of psychiatric diagnoses. In particular, this chapter has proposed that a recognition of how psychiatric diagnosis is made against a background of such values and norms challenges the way in which that practice seeks to legitimise itself as being concerned with the identification of naturally occurring biologically based medical disorders. Finally, we have concluded by considering an alternative to psychiatric diagnosis that has been most closely associated with the discipline of clinical psychology and is commonly referred to as psychological formulation or simply formulation. Comparing this approach to psychiatric diagnosis, this chapter has examined how the thoughts, feelings and behaviours that are associated with mental distress can be understood as meaningful once they are considered, through the use of formulation, in the unique context of a person's life history and current circumstances.

ACTIVITIES: BRIEF OUTLINE ANSWERS

ACTIVITY 3.1 RESEARCH

In conducting your own investigations into Rosenhan's study you should have discovered that by seeking to investigate the ability of mental health professionals to distinguish 'normality' from 'abnormality', Rosenhan and seven other volunteers presented themselves at various mental health hospitals stating that they had been hearing a voice saying 'empty', 'hollow' and 'thud'. Immediately after admission, all eight volunteers or 'pseudo-patients' stopped simulating any further symptoms of mental distress and for the remainder of their time in hospital behaved as they would have normally behaved. Despite this normal behaviour, the mental health professionals in the various hospital settings never reported any concerns that the volunteers were in fact pseudo-patients. Instead, all but one of the volunteers received a diagnosis of schizophrenia and all were discharged from hospital with a diagnosis of 'schizophrenia in remission'.

In considering the implications of this, Rosenhan suggested that the mental health professionals were operating with the powerful assumption that all of the people who had been admitted to the hospital were 'abnormal' in various ways and this assumption led them to either overlook or misinterpret everyday normal behaviours. For example, walking the hospital corridors to alleviate boredom was interpreted as possible 'nervousness'; writing things down was understood as the potentially compulsive expression of some form of psychological disturbance; and being seated outside the cafeteria entrance half an hour before lunchtime was understood as an 'oral-acquisitive syndrome' (Rosenhan 1973, p. 253). Therefore, rather than being able to distinguish normality from abnormality, Rosenhan's study powerfully illustrated how the diagnostic judgements of mental health professionals can be profoundly influenced by the environment in which those judgements are made. In particular, it highlights how mental health settings, and clinical environments in general, can lead practitioners to make unwarranted and distorted assumptions about the behaviour of the people who are temporarily situated there.

ACTIVITY 3.2 REFLECTION

In considering how Khanyi's thoughts, feelings and behaviours might be more productively understood as meaningful responses to, and strategies for coping with, adverse life events and challenging circumstances, you might have identified how it would be necessary to situate her experiences within the unique context of her life. However, while you ought to be cautious about making any generalisations about the factors that contribute to mental distress, there is evidence to suggest that a significant number of people who are diagnosed with borderline personality disorder have a history of experiencing childhood trauma such as emotional, sexual and violent physical abuse (Zanarini & Wedig 2014; Fetridge et al. 2015).

While it would be necessary to consider such findings in the context of Khanyi's unique circumstances and life history, you may have considered how her displays of anger and aggression, her feelings of guilt and powerlessness and the value she appears to place on loyalty, trust and security might be responses to previous experiences of trauma and abuse. Moreover, you may have considered how Khanyi's repeated engagement in self-harm behaviours and her possible 'dissociative' experiences (reflected in her sense of detachment and feeling as though she 'doesn't really exist') might be understood as strategies to address feelings of powerless-ness and achieve a degree of control and self-determination over her life (Proctor 2007).

ACTIVITY 3.3 TEAM WORKING

In attempting to provide a provisional team formulation for Dylan's experience of mental dis-tress, and his unusual beliefs in particular, you may have suggested that such a process would in practice necessitate his full participation in order to explore his understanding of that experi-ence. However, from the information given about his life history and his current circumstances, you might have had interesting discussions with your colleagues about the factors that may have contributed to the emergence and the maintenance of his mental distress. For example, you might have discussed how the violence that he was subjected to as a child, his mother's dismissal of his reports of its occurrence and the manner in which it influenced his beliefs about how to deal with difficulties and the extent to which others can be trusted may have been predisposing factors for the emergence of his mental distress and his unusual beliefs about his co-workers.

In addition, you might have discussed how Dylan's experiences may have been precipitated by the competitive atmosphere in his work environment, how he responded by consistently working late, the serious argument with his work colleagues and how these factors have inter-acted with his distrust of others. Moreover, you might have suggested that his mental distress may be being perpetuated by the character of his work environment, his apparent social iso-lation and his enduring belief about keeping his difficulties to himself. Finally, in considering those factors that might alleviate Dylan's mental distress or prevent its recurrence, you may have identified the need to address the challenges and conflict in his work environment, to maintain the social support from his sister and his friends and to help Dylan reconsider the value of retaining his beliefs about how to deal with difficulties and the extent to which others can be trusted.

FURTHER READING

- **Johnstone L** (2014) *A Straight Talking Introduction to Psychiatric Diagnosis.* Ross-on-Wye: PCCS Books.

An accessible introduction to a variety of critical issues surrounding psychiatric diagnosis which includes a discussion of the multiple negative consequences that can be associated with receiving such a diagnosis.

- **Johnstone L & Dallos R** (eds) (2014) *Formulation in Psychology and Psychotherapy: Making Sense of People's Problems*, 2nd edition. Hove: Routledge.

This is a comprehensive account of the theoretical and practical issues surrounding the use of formulation in understanding mental distress that examines its use from a variety of therapeutic perspectives.

- **Szasz T** (1983) The myth of mental illness. In Szasz T, *Ideology and Insanity: Essays on the Psychiatric Dehumanization of Man.* London: Marion Boyars.

Here you will find the classic critical discussion of the role that social, cultural and historical values and norms have in the identification of mental distress by one of the most provocative and controversial figures in psychiatry.

- **Watters E** (2011) *Crazy Like Us: The Globalization of the Western Mind.* London: Constable & Robinson.

This is a stimulating book that examines the social, cultural and historical values that are inherent in Western ideas of mental distress, and which also considers how these values and ideas are being 'exported' to other cultures around the world.

USEFUL WEBSITES

- www.psychdiagnosis.weebly.com

Here you will find a website that explores the consequences of psychiatric diagnoses for those who receive them and provides multiple videos and stories of the harm that people have experienced as a result.

- www.psychiatry.org/psychiatrists/practice/dsm

This is the website for the American Psychiatric Association that provides a variety of resources about the *Diagnostic and Statistical Manual of Mental Disorders*, including details about its latest edition and its diagnostic categories.

PSYCHIATRIC DRUGS

CHAPTER AIMS

By the end of this chapter you will be able to:

- evaluate the disease-centred model of how psychiatric drugs work;
- appraise the alternative drug-centred model of how psychiatric drugs work;
- assess the implications of these two models for mental health care.

INTRODUCTION

CASE STUDY

Deon is a 32-year-old man who was given a diagnosis of schizophrenia in his early twenties and has since had multiple mental health hospital admissions. Several days ago he was readmitted to hospital after a deterioration in his mental state which coincided with the breakdown of his relationship with his long-term partner. Since being on the ward the staff have reported that Deon has been 'responding to auditory hallucinations' and that he has also been experiencing 'sleep disturbances'. This has meant that he has been awake throughout the night and has spent large parts of the day in bed. Following assessment by a psychiatrist, Deon has been prescribed an antipsychotic drug in addition to the one that he is currently prescribed. Over the past several days, however, the staff have observed that he is becoming increasingly anxious, restless and has displayed what they refer to as 'threatening behaviour'. In response to these reports, Deon has also been prescribed the short-acting benzodiazepine lorazepam which is to be used by the staff when they feel it is necessary.

Ever since the introduction of chlorpromazine in the 1950s, psychiatric drugs have commonly been presented as revolutionising the treatment of mental distress. They have been credited with enabling people to leave institutionalised hospital care and reclaim productive lives in the community, of breaking links with outmoded and inhumane forms of treatment and with placing mental health care on the same scientific foundation that is said to characterise other branches of modern medicine (Shorter 1997; Lieberman 2016). This perception of psychiatric drugs has, in part, contributed to their widespread use in contemporary mental health care and, as illustrated in the above case study, become the intervention that people experiencing mental distress are often most likely to receive. However, despite the centrality of the use of a wide range of psychiatric drugs in mental health care (Table 4.1), there exists a variety of critical debates surrounding this form of intervention. For example, there are critical questions about the degree to which the suggested benefits of psychiatric drugs outweigh the range of adverse effects that they can produce, both short term and long term. There are also ongoing concerns about various prescribing practices such as **polypharmacy**, the use of excessive or 'megadoses' of certain classes of psychiatric drugs and the extent to which people who take those drugs are involved in decisions about their use. In addition, there are critical discussions about the quality of the research into the efficacy of psychiatric drugs and, in particular, provocative analyses of the influence of the pharmaceutical industry on such research (Breggin 1993; Bentall 2010; Gøtzsche 2013).

The purpose of this chapter is to introduce you to a variety of critical issues surrounding the use of psychiatric drugs and the manner in which they are thought to work. While being infrequently articulated, ideas about how psychiatric drugs are thought to work are central to a variety of critical debates in contemporary mental health care, including the way in which psychiatric drugs are used, the manner in which their potential benefits are balanced against their adverse effects and the extent to which those who use psychiatric drugs are meaningfully involved in decisions about their use. This chapter will therefore begin by examining the widespread

Table 4.1 Psychiatric drug classification

Class	Subclass	Example (UK and US generic and trade names)
Antipsychotics	First generation or 'typical' Second generation or 'atypical'	Chlorpromazine (Largactil/Thorazine) Olanzapine (Zyprexa)
Antidepressants	Selective serotonin reuptake inhibitors (SSRIs)	Fluoxetine (Prozac)
	Serotonin and noradrenaline reuptake inhibitors (SNRIs)	Venlafaxine (Effexor)
	Tricyclic antidepressants	Trimipramine (Surmontil)
	Monoamine oxidase inbibitors (MAOIs)	Phenelzine (Nardil)
	Other antidepressants	Agomelatine (Valdoxan)
Mood stabilisers	Lithium	Lithium carbonate (Camcolit/Eskalith)
	Anticonvulsants	Carbamazepine (Tegretol)
	Antipsychotics	Risperidone (Risperdal)
Anxiolytics	Benzodiazepines	Diazepam (Valium)
	SSRIs	Sertraline (Lustral/Zoloft)
	S1 agonists	Buspirone (Buspar)
Stimulants		Methylphenidate (Ritalin)

although often implicitly held belief that psychiatric drugs work by targeting and correcting the biological dysfunctions or chemical imbalances that supposedly underlie the emergence and maintenance of mental distress. However, rather than understanding psychiatric drugs as precise medications or 'magic bullets' that target and correct chemical imbalances, we shall then discuss an alternative conception of how psychiatric drugs work. This alternative way of thinking about psychiatric drugs suggests that they are powerful psychoactive substances that produce a range of altered states and non-specific physiological and psychological effects. Finally, this chapter will examine the implications of these two pharmacological models for how psychiatric drugs are used in contemporary mental health care and for the character of the clinical and therapeutic relationship between mental health professionals and those who use psychiatric drugs.

THE DISEASE-CENTRED MODEL OF PSYCHIATRIC DRUGS

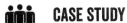 **CASE STUDY**

Malina is in the fifth week of her clinical placement on a forensic mental health unit and her mentor, Samuel, is providing her with feedback about her knowledge of psychiatric medication. Samuel is impressed with Malina's knowledge of both the generic and trade names for common drugs used in psychiatry and also to which class each of those individual drugs belong. However, Malina is keen to deepen her knowledge about all aspects of psychiatric medication and asks her mentor how psychiatric drugs work. Samuel replies that they work by acting on the specific chemical imbalances and biological dysfunctions that are associated with mental distress and which give rise to the particular symptoms that people experience. He suggests that how psychiatric drugs work is reflected in the names that are used to classify those drugs. So, for example, the drugs that target the chemical imbalances that lead to depression are called 'antidepressants', the drugs that correct the biological mechanisms that cause psychosis are called 'antipsychotics' and the drugs that act upon the underlying dysfunctions that lead to mood instability are called 'mood stabilisers'.

In the case study above, Malina's mentor is expressing the widely held belief that psychiatric drugs work by acting upon the supposed biological dysfunctions and disease processes that are often presented as being implicated in the emergence and maintenance of mental distress. This explanation of how psychiatric drugs work draws upon a general pharmacological model, referred to as the **disease-centred model**, that is used to explain how drugs in other fields of modern medicine are understood as targeting the biological causes of a disease or the biological processes that produce the symptoms associated with a particular disease (Moncrieff 2008). For example, in explaining how psychiatric drugs work by drawing upon this disease-centred model, those drugs are sometimes presented as working in a way that is broadly analogous to how insulin works in diabetes.

That is, in a manner somewhat similar to how insulin alleviates the symptoms associated with diabetes by compensating for the body's inability to produce sufficient quantities of that hormone, psychiatric drugs are sometimes presented as alleviating and even eliminating the symptoms associated with mental distress by targeting and correcting the biological dysfunctions that are claimed to cause such distress. For example, in highlighting the supposedly precise and targeted character of the psychiatric drugs that emerged during the 1950s in comparison with previous interventions for mental distress, it has been suggested that 'What made chlorpromazine, imipramine, and lithium so different from the sedatives and tranquilizers that came before was that they directly targeted psychiatric symptoms in a kind of lock-and-key relationship' (Lieberman 2016, p. 188).

In the context of this disease-centred model, the biological dysfunction that is most commonly invoked as being implicated in the emergence and maintenance of mental distress, and which psychiatric drugs are said to target and correct, are chemical imbalances in the brain. Indeed, the manner in which psychiatric drugs have been found to exert an influence upon the action of a variety of neurotransmitters (the chemicals that are involved in the transmission of information between the neurons that make up the brain) has often been invoked as evidence for the suggestion that mental distress is a consequence of some form of chemical imbalance. For example, antipsychotic drugs have been found to block the action of the neurotransmitter dopamine and this has been used to formulate, and as evidence to support, the dopamine hypothesis of schizophrenia. While various versions of this hypothesis have been presented, in its most general sense it maintains that the experiences associated with a diagnosis of schizophrenia arise as a consequence of some form of imbalance in, and in particular an over-stimulation of, the neurotransmitter dopamine (Howes & Kapur 2009). Similarly, many antidepressant drugs are understood to inhibit the reuptake of serotonin and noradrenaline, both classed as monoamine neurotransmitters, and this has been used to formulate, and as evidence to support, the monoamine hypothesis of depression. In doing so, it has been suggested that the experiences associated with a diagnosis of depression are a manifestation of some form of imbalance in, and in particular a deficiency of, either serotonin or noradrenaline, or a combination of these two neurotransmitters (Hirschfeld 2000; Mulinari 2012).

CONCEPT SUMMARY: THE NEUROCHEMICAL SELF

The notion that the experiences associated with mental distress are a consequence of some form of neurochemical imbalance, an imbalance that can be addressed by drugs that are supposedly designed to target and correct such neurochemical dysfunctions, has become a pervasive way to understand and respond to those experiences. However, the employment of such neurochemical explanations is not confined to the field of mental health care. Rather, it has been suggested that our everyday thoughts, feelings and behaviours are increasingly understood in terms our neurochemistry, and this trend reflects a more widespread transformation throughout contemporary

Western societies in which professionals from a diversity of disciplines have come 'to understand our minds and selves in terms of our brains and bodies' (Rose 2003, p. 46).

Moreover, this tendency to reframe aspects of human experience in biochemical terms, and an associated tendency to seek to modify that experience through the employment of a variety of chemical compounds, is not confined to the professional domain. Rather, it has been suggested that individuals themselves are increasingly disposed 'to recode their moods and their ills in terms of the functioning of their brain chemicals, and to act upon themselves in the light of this belief' (Rose 2003, p. 59). As a consequence, contemporary Western societies are said to be undergoing a profound 'neurochemical reframing of the self' and a 'pharmacological reshaping of society' in which the theoretical understanding of human experience in biochemical terms, and the practical modification of that experience by pharmaceutical means, is becoming increasingly routine.

Despite its pervasiveness both within and beyond the field of mental health care, the suggestion that various types of chemical imbalance are implicated in mental distress, and that psychiatric drugs work by acting upon these imbalances, has been a matter of ongoing critical consideration. In particular, such claims have been subject to sustained criticism from a variety of perspectives, with detailed discussions of, for example, the social, economic and political factors that have contributed to the emergence of this way of understanding mental distress and the drugs used to respond to that distress (Double 2011; Lacasse & Leo 2015; Whitaker 2015). Arguably the most fundamental critique, however, is the suggestion that there is a lack of reliable, replicable and therefore compelling evidence for any form of biological dysfunction in mental distress, including any form of chemical imbalance. As highlighted in Chapter 2, a clear and convincing biological cause has not been demonstrated for the vast majority of 'psychiatric disorders', including schizophrenia, bipolar disorder and depression (Cromby *et al.* 2013; Deacon 2013). Indeed, while it is common to encounter claims that mental distress is a consequence of some form of chemical imbalance, and that psychiatric drugs work by specifically acting upon these imbalances, it has variously been suggested that the evidence for such claims is unconvincing, misleading or simply non-existent (Moncrieff 2008; Gøtzsche 2013; Lynch 2015).

To propose that there is no compelling evidence to justify the assertion that various forms of chemical imbalance are implicated in mental distress, imbalances that psychiatric drugs selectively target and address, may strike some as a controversial claim. It seems intuitively correct to conclude that because psychiatric drugs can have beneficial effects upon the various symptoms associated with mental distress, and that those drugs act upon an individual's neurochemisty in certain ways, then those symptoms must have been the result of some form of dysfunction or imbalance in that neurochemistry. However, while such arguments are commonplace and seem intuitively plausible, the form of thinking that they involve (what is referred to as *ex juvantibus* reasoning) is insufficient by itself to establish that the symptoms associated with mental distress are a consequence of some form of neurochemical dysfunction. Indeed, there are many instances in which drugs can produce beneficial effects upon the symptoms associated with a variety of conditions, and do so by modifying an individual's biological systems in particular ways, and yet those systems play no part in the emergence of those conditions (Busfield 2011). For example, aspirin and paracetamol can alleviate the symptoms associated with a variety of conditions, including influenza and migraines; however, the fact that they achieve these effects by modifying biological systems in particular ways does not mean that such conditions are caused by dysfunctions or imbalances in the systems upon which aspirin and paracetamol act (Lacasse & Leo 2005; Rose 2006).

PRACTICE ISSUE: ANTIDEPRESSANTS AND THE PLACEBO EFFECT

The effectiveness of antidepressants in alleviating the symptoms associated with depression is commonly invoked to support the assertion that such drugs act upon a supposed chemical imbalance that underlies those symptoms. Therefore, if antidepressants worked by correcting a chemical imbalance, somewhat similar to how insulin works in diabetes, then we would expect those drugs to be significantly more effective than a **placebo**. However, while the available evidence indicates that antidepressants are more effective than a placebo in the treatment of depression, it has been suggested that this effect is so small that those drugs cannot be considered as possessing a 'clinically significant advantage' over a placebo (Kirsch 2014, p. 129).

Indeed, rather than correcting some supposed chemical imbalance, the minimal advantage that antidepressants have over a placebo has been attributed to methodological issues related to the research process. For example, in trials that compare antidepressants with a placebo, the participants initially do not know whether they have received the former or the latter such that they are 'blind' to which intervention they are receiving. However, it has been suggested that many participants in such trials are able to detect if they are taking the active drug or the placebo and one of the reasons given for this is that those receiving the active drug will begin to experience the adverse effects produced by that drug (Rabkin et al. 1986; Even et al. 2000).

It has therefore been proposed that the minimal advantage that antidepressants have over placebo in clinical trials is not attributable to their supposedly antidepressant properties and, in particular, their ability to address some supposed neurochemical imbalance. Rather, it is said to be a consequence of how participants in those trials 'break the blind' and detect that they are taking an antidepressant rather than a placebo, which can thereby create the powerful expectation in the participants that the drug will help. As Kirsch (2011) has suggested, 'it is possible that the superiority of active antidepressant to inert placebo is due to the breaking of blind by patients in the active drug condition. Rather than being a true drug effect, it is an enhanced placebo effect' (p. 192).

If there is a lack of compelling evidence to support claims that mental distress is a consequence of some form of chemical imbalance, and that psychiatric drugs work by addressing those imbalances, the question arises as to how they have been able to proliferate both within and beyond mental health care. As we have previously highlighted, the reasons why any one particular way of understanding and responding to mental distress becomes influential are complex and cannot simply be attributed to a supposed theoretical and therapeutic superiority over other approaches. Indeed, the enduring influence of neurochemical explanations for mental distress and the conception of psychiatric drugs as 'chemical cures' have been attributed to a variety of social, political and economic factors (Moncrieff 2008; Busfield 2015; Whitaker 2015). For example, it has been suggested that the pharmaceutical industry, driven by a financial imperative to maximise profits, has relentlessly employed various marketing strategies to promote chemical imbalance theories of mental distress and the effectiveness of psychiatric drugs to address those imbalances. Moreover, the proliferation of such claims has been attributed to the way in which they provide a seductively accessible account of how to understand mental distress which has therefore been readily perpetuated throughout society by, for example, the mass media. In addition, it has been proposed that such claims are politically expedient in so far as they divert attention away from a consideration of the wider social and material conditions that can contribute to mental distress, as well as the more financially and politically demanding task of addressing those conditions.

One of the most challenging proposals, however, is that mental health professionals have been instrumental in proliferating the notion that mental distress is a manifestation of some form of chemical imbalance that psychiatric drugs are able to address. The reasons for their doing so have variously been attributed to an unfamiliarity with the available research on psychiatric drugs, to deficiencies in the education and training of mental health professionals, and to a desire on the part of practitioners and the various professions to which they belong to be perceived as possessing treatments that are analogous to those used in other branches of medicine (Moncrieff 2015). However, one of the most disturbing suggestions is that mental health professionals have employed chemical imbalance theories as 'productive metaphors' in order to achieve a range of clinical objectives (Lacasse & Leo 2015). For example, it has been proposed that such explanations have been used to provide people with an accessible account of the complex, confusing and sometimes disturbing experiences that can be associated with mental distress. In addition, it has been suggested that claims about the precise and targeted character of psychiatric drugs have been sustained in order to reassure people that practitioners, when they prescribe and administer those drugs, have a sophisticated understanding of how they work. Moreover, there are even suggestions that mental health professionals have perpetuated notions that psychiatric drugs address the chemical imbalances of which mental distress is a supposed manifestation in order to facilitate confidence in the effectiveness of psychiatric drugs as a response to that distress (Lacasse & Leo 2015).

CONCEPT SUMMARY: THE PHARMACEUTICAL INDUSTRY

The role of the pharmaceutical industry in contemporary mental health care, and the influence it has on shaping how mental distress is understood and addressed, has been the subject of sustained critique. In broad terms, the pharmaceutical industry is concerned with developing treatments for health problems, and it has been suggested that not only have some of the drugs it has developed (such as antibiotics, analgesics and antihistamines) undoubtedly been of value, but that the industry also has an important role in promoting health and well-being (Busfield 2015). However, it is important to recognise that the pharmaceutical industry is a powerful global industry, made up of a small number of large, multinational companies, whose primary aim is to maintain and increase the financial profits of the products that it develops. It is this drive to maximise profits, and the various practices that it engages in to pursue that objective, which forms the basis of many of the critical issues surrounding the influence of the pharmaceutical industry in mental health care.

Studies into the efficacy of psychiatric drugs are increasingly being funded by the pharmaceutical industry, and it has been suggested that, in comparison with independently sponsored trials, the industry is more likely to report the effectiveness of its drugs while minimising and even concealing their harmful effects (Gøtzsche 2013; Healey 2014). In addition, the marketing practices of drug companies and the inducements to encourage practitioners to prescribe their products have been the target of criticism, with such inducements ranging from small gifts bearing the brand name of a drug through to substantial financial remuneration for acting as a pharmaceutical company consultant (Bentall 2010). Moreover, it has been suggested that the industry not only engages in a variety of activities to promote a biological understanding of mental distress and exclude alternative approaches, it also expands the existing boundaries of what is considered a mental health problem and even contributes to the establishment of new psychiatric diagnoses in order to create markets for its products (Busfield 2015; Whitaker & Cosgrove 2015).

THE DRUG-CENTRED MODEL OF PSYCHIATRIC DRUGS

👥 CASE STUDY

Although David has recently been diagnosed with social anxiety disorder, he can recall having a fear of social situations and interacting with others at least since adolescence. Following discussion with his general practitioner about the degree to which his social anxiety is increasingly causing problems with various aspects of his daily life, David was prescribed an SSRI. Although he felt less anxious while he was taking that psychiatric drug, he began to experience a range of adverse physical effects (such as stomach upsets, insomnia and sexual problems) and subsequently stopped taking it. As an alternative strategy to attempt to deal with his social anxiety, David has begun to use moderate amounts of alcohol. While he has found that using alcohol has led to some unwanted effects, most notably a disruption in the quality of his sleep, its use has also alleviated many of the physical symptoms associated with his experiences of social anxiety (including nausea, sweating and palpitations) and this has helped him to interact with others in social situations in a less self-conscious way.

In so far as the disease-centred model of psychiatric drugs has been subject to sustained criticism from a variety of perspectives, an alternative pharmacological model has been proposed by which to understand the action of those drugs. In contrast to the disease-centred model, this alternative **drug-centred model** maintains that psychiatric drugs do not work by acting upon and addressing some supposed chemical imbalance that contributes to the emergence and maintenance of mental distress (Moncrieff 2008). Rather, the drug-centred model proposes that psychiatric drugs are powerful **psychoactive substances** that act upon the central nervous system to produce various alterations in a person's thoughts, feelings and behaviour. Therefore, while the disease-centred model of psychiatric drugs is often illustrated by claiming that those drugs work in a way that is similar to how insulin works in diabetes, the drug-centred model can be illustrated by the way in which alcohol is used by some people to help with certain experiences associated with mental distress. In the above case study, for example, David has begun to experience a range of symptoms associated with a diagnosis of social anxiety disorder and he has discovered that a moderate use of alcohol has been helpful in dealing with those symptoms. However, alcohol is not here understood in a disease-centred way as targeting and correcting some supposed chemical imbalance that is causing David's mental distress. Instead, it is understood in a drug-centred way as acting upon the central nervous system to produce an altered state and a range of physiological and psychological effects, some of which David has found helpful in dealing with his social anxiety.

Rather than being magic bullets that selectively target and correct some form of chemical imbalance or biological dysfunction that supposedly underlies mental distress, the drug-centred model therefore maintains that psychiatric drugs are imprecise substances or 'blunt instruments'. In particular, this pharmacological model proposes that psychiatric drugs are powerful psychoactive substances that act upon the central nervous system in a global rather than a precise manner, and by doing so they change or 'perturb' normal neurotransmitter function to produce a range of altered mental and physical states (Hyman & Nestler 1996; Whitaker 2015). Therefore, while the disease-centred model suggests that psychiatric drugs work by returning supposedly imbalanced, dysfunctional and abnormal brain states back to normal, the drug-based model maintains that psychiatric drugs produce abnormal, artificial or intoxicated brain states by disrupting normal neurotransmitter function (Breggin 2006; Moncrieff 2015). In this pharmacological model, each psychiatric drug is understood as producing its own distinctive drug-induced state that has a variety of physiological and psychological effects, effects that may be experienced by some people as being helpful in dealing with the symptoms that can be associated with mental distress. In illustrating this drug-centred understanding of psychiatric drugs, and the manner in which the altered states that those drugs produce may be experienced by some people as beneficial, Moncrieff (2013) makes it clear that 'The drug-centred model suggests that drugs can sometimes be helpful because the features of the altered drug-induced state superimpose themselves onto the manifestations of distress' (p. 161).

Table 4.2 Pharmacological models of how psychiatric drugs work (Moncrieff 2015)

Disease-centred model	Drug-centred model
Psychiatric drugs are magic bullets	Psychiatric drugs are blunt instruments
Psychiatric drugs correct an abnormal brain state	Psychiatric drugs create an abnormal brain state
Beneficial effects arise from the correction of chemical imbalances	Beneficial effects arise from the creation of drug-induced states
Commonly illustrated with the example of the use of insulin for diabetes	Commonly illustrated with the example of the use of alcohol for social anxiety

In order to further understand how the drug-centred model maintains that psychiatric drugs can produce effects that some people may find beneficial, it is productive to examine that model in the context of the use of antipsychotic drugs. As a response to the experiences associated with a diagnosis of schizophrenia, these drugs are not to be understood as correcting some form of imbalance in a person's neurochemistry, such as an overstimulation of dopamine. Rather, by blocking the action of dopamine and affecting a range of other brain systems, the drug-centred model suggests that antipsychotics create a drug-induced state similar to Parkinson's disease in which mental and physical activity is suppressed – a condition which has variously been referred to as a state of 'deactivation', 'immobilisation' or 'tranquilisation' (Breggin 1993; Moncrieff 2008; Healey 2016). This tranquilised state, however, should not be thought of as being comparable to a condition of relaxation, and neither should it be thought of as some form of 'chemical cosh or straightjacket' – although antipsychotics can produce a state of immobilised sedation if used in high enough doses (Bentall 2010, p. 221). Instead, antipsychotics are said to produce a state of indifference or detachment, a 'who cares feeling' that some may find helpful for the so-called **positive symptoms** of schizophrenia by suppressing, or making people less responsive to, the presence of hallucinations, delusions and the anxiety that can accompany them (Mizrahi *et al.* 2005; Kapur *et al.* 2006).

Rather than being a chemical cure that removes the distressing experiences associated with schizophrenia, the drug-centred model therefore maintains that antipsychotics produce an altered state in which people can become less concerned by those experiences. However, although some people may find those drugs beneficial in this way, it is important to recognise that the general suppression of mental and physical activity that they produce does not selectively target particular experiences associated with schizophrenia (Barnes 2011). That is, while creating a distinctive state of indifference or detachment, antipsychotics do not simply create a sense of detachment from the experiences associated with a diagnosis of schizophrenia, but can also create a sense of indifference towards all experiences. For example, those who use antipsychotics report that the full range of human emotions can not only come to be experienced with less intensity, but there can be an emotional flattening or blunting that is characterised by a lack or absence of emotion (Moncrieff *et al.* 2015; Healey 2016). Similarly, the generalised suppression of mental and physical activity that antipsychotics produce may not only impair a person's attention, memory and general thought processes, but it can also reduce their motivation to initiate actions, carry out simple tasks and engage with others. Indeed, such effects can present as being similar to the so-called **negative symptoms** of schizophrenia (which include apathy, social withdrawal and reduced motivation), and it has been suggested that it is unclear how the state of deactivation or tranquilisation that antipsychotics produce can assist in the alleviation of these symptoms.

──────── **PRACTICE ISSUE: ATYPICAL ANTIPSYCHOTICS** ────────

It is commonly claimed that the newer second generation or 'atypical' antipsychotics are superior in a variety of ways to the older first generation or 'typical' antipsychotics in the treatment of schizophrenia and psychosis. However, with the exception of clozapine (which is indicated in 'treatment-resistant schizophrenia') atypical antipsychotics have not been found to be more effective in alleviating the positive symptoms of schizophrenia, and both typical and atypical antipsychotics show limited benefit for the treatment of negative symptoms (Erhart *et al.* 2006; Lewis & Lieberman 2008). Moreover, while there are no accepted criteria for the classification of an antipsychotic as atypical, the term is often associated with claims that this class of antipsychotics produces fewer adverse effects and fewer **extrapyramidal effects** in particular.

There is evidence to suggest, however, that there is no substantial difference in the production of extrapyramidal effects between typical and atypical antipsychotics (Jones *et al.* 2006; Miller *et al.* 2008; Moore & Furberg 2016). Therefore, it has been proposed that it is unproductive to think of these drugs as belonging to two distinct groups, with one producing fewer adverse effects (Kendall 2011; Leucht *et al.* 2013; Parker 2013). Indeed, while all antipsychotics can produce adverse effects, atypical antipsychotics have been associated with an increased risk of metabolic syndrome (a cluster of conditions including obesity, hyperlipidaemia and hyperglycaemia), which increases the risk of cardiovascular disease and is one of the leading causes of morbidity and mortality in those with a diagnosis of schizophrenia (Pramyothin & Khaodhiar 2010; Riordan *et al.* 2011).

While the drug-centred model illustrates how psychiatric drugs can produce altered states and a range of physiological and psychological effects that some people may find beneficial, it also helps to understand how those drugs can produce a range of undesirable, adverse effects. As powerful psychoactive substances that act upon the central nervous system to alter normal functioning in a global rather than a targeted way, psychiatric drugs (in a manner similar to alcohol) can produce a range of effects that may not only be unpleasant and unhelpful but can also contribute to the risk of physical morbidity and mortality (Correll *et al.* 2015). However, while psychiatric drugs can produce a variety of adverse effects, it has been suggested that mental health professionals may be unaware of the full range of those effects, and can minimise their significance for the person taking the drug or misinterpret such effects as a deterioration in a person's mental health rather than as adverse reactions caused by the psychiatric drug (Breggin 2006; Read 2009). Indeed, it has been proposed that there can be a tendency in mental health settings to attribute a deterioration in a person's well-being to a relapse or worsening of their 'underlying mental disorder' rather than to an adverse effect produced by a psychiatric drug; as a consequence, there can be a demand to respond to such a perceived deterioration or relapse by increasing the dosages of psychiatric drugs, which, in turn, can increase the risks of adverse drug reactions (Healey 2016).

In order to provide informed, safe and effective mental health care that is responsive to the needs of people who use mental health services, it has been suggested that practitioners should develop their ability to recognise the range of adverse effects, both short term and long term, that psychiatric drugs can produce (Healey 2016). Doing so, however, can be a considerable challenge. The briefest of investigations will reveal that psychiatric drugs have been associated with an extensive, surprising and alarming range of adverse effects. These will not only include predictable adverse effects that are caused by the drugs' normal pharmacological activity, such as the extrapyramidal effects associated with antipsychotics or the risk of toxicity associated with lithium; rather, psychiatric drugs can also produce a range of idiosyncratic, unpredictable effects that result from processes not yet fully understood and that may go largely unrecognised, such as the **serotonin syndrome** associated with antidepressants and selective serotonin reuptake inhibitors in particular (Ellahi 2015). To facilitate the reporting and recognition of the range of adverse effects that can be produced by psychiatric drugs, it has therefore been suggested that it is necessary to create a clinical climate in which those taking such drugs feel able to report potential adverse drug reactions. Central to achieving this is a willingness on the part of mental health professionals to remain open-minded about the possibility that any problems reported, even those that are not generally considered to be established or predictable adverse effects, may be a consequence of taking a psychiatric drug (Healey 2016).

ACTIVITY 4.1   RESEARCH

It has been suggested that akathisia is potentially one of the most serious adverse effects that can be produced by psychiatric drugs. While it is commonly associated with the use of antipsychotics, it is increasingly being recognised as an adverse effect associated with the use of antidepressants (Healey 2016).

For this activity conduct your own investigations into drug-induced akathisia and the characteristic features of that adverse drug effect. As you do so, attempt to provide a brief overview of the observable movements associated with that condition as well as a sense of akathisia as a subjective experience.

An outline answer is provided at the end of the chapter.

THE PRACTICE IMPLICATIONS OF PSYCHIATRIC DRUG MODELS

ᎦᎦᎦ CASE STUDY

Louise is a mental health professional who is currently visiting Kadir after he was discharged home following his six-month admission to an acute mental health hospital. While he is currently taking the psychiatric drugs that are prescribed for him, Kadir has told Louise that he has started to think about discontinuing the additional drug that he commenced in hospital because he feels that he no longer needs it and that it is causing various unwanted effects. Louise has replied that while the effects that he is experiencing may be a consequence of the new drug, it is important that he continues to adhere to the drug regime that was formulated for him. She has suggested that the psychiatric drugs he is taking are helping to support his recovery by preventing a recurrence of his symptoms and a potential readmission to hospital. While Louise acknowledges that the 'side-effects' that the drug may be causing can be 'unpleasant', she also suggests that these are outweighed by the benefits that the psychiatric drugs are having upon his mental health.

The enduring influence of the disease-centred model of psychiatric drugs can be understood as having far-reaching implications for the people who take those drugs and for the manner in which they are used in contemporary mental health care. In so far as psychiatric drugs have been understood as precise medications or magic bullets that target and correct some form of chemical imbalance or biological dysfunction, then decisions about those drugs (such as dose, duration and discontinuation) have largely come to be seen as technical matters that are determined by mental health professionals. As a consequence, the experiences and opinions of those who use psychiatric drugs have commonly been subordinated to the specialist knowledge and judgements of practitioners. While there is an emerging interest in equitable, shared decision-making between mental health professionals and those who use mental health services with respect to psychiatric drugs, it has been suggested that the meaningful involvement of people who use those drugs in decisions about their use remains, in practice, limited (Matthias *et al.* 2012; Kaminskiy *et al.* 2013; Morant *et al.* 2016). Indeed, as illustrated in the above case study, the relationship between mental health professionals and those who use psychiatric drugs can become centred around the issue of 'medication adherence'. Often as a consequence of poor 'compliance' on the part of those prescribed psychiatric drugs, practitioners can become focused upon attempting to ensure that people experiencing mental distress adhere to the drug regimes that have been formulated for them (Deegan & Drake 2006).

By maintaining both the short- and long-term effectiveness of psychiatric drugs to support a person's recovery, and to prevent future episodes of mental distress, practitioners can employ a range of strategies to ensure medication compliance (Mitchell & Selmes 2007; Chapman & Horne 2013). While recommendations are often made that compliance should occur in the context of a therapeutic alliance, it has been claimed that it is also secured through the use of various forms of coercion such as 'subtle persuasion', 'strategic dishonesty' and compulsory enforcement of drug treatment (Seale *et al.* 2006; Chaplin 2007). For example, in an attempt to ensure compliance with psychiatric medication, the experience of the adverse effects of those drugs can be given minimal consideration by mental health professionals. Indeed, when adverse effects are reported by those using psychiatric drugs, it has been suggested that practitioners have been found to contest, disbelieve or disregard those reports (Seale *et al.* 2007; Read 2009). Moreover, in so far as psychiatric drugs are understood as targeting and correcting some form of chemical imbalance or biological dysfunction there is an implicit assumption about the effectiveness of their use. As illustrated in the above case study, this can manifest itself in the way in which any negative consequences of using a psychiatric drug are referred to as 'side' effects that, while potentially 'unpleasant', are seen as tolerable by-products of a drug's supposedly beneficial 'main' effects of correcting the dysfunctions that are thought to cause mental distress (Moncrieff & Cohen 2009).

PRACTICE ISSUE: THE DISCONTINUATION EFFECT

The evidence base for the effectiveness of psychiatric drugs to prevent the recurrence of mental distress, and therefore to be used on a long-term basis, has been subject to critical debate and dispute. For example, it has variously been suggested that the benefits have been exaggerated, the adverse effects underestimated, and there has been an overly narrow focus on the ability of psychiatric drugs to prevent the recurrence of symptoms rather than help people to recover meaningful psychological and social functioning (Double 2011; Wunderink *et al.* 2013; Gøtzsche *et al.* 2015).

It has also been argued that a potential methodological problem with the evidence-base for the long-term use of psychiatric drugs has been a failure to account for what has been referred to as the **discontinuation effect**. To understand this methodological issue it is productive to note that the evidence for the effectiveness of the long-term use of psychiatric drugs has often derived from studies that involve selecting people who have been taking those drugs on a long-term basis and then randomly assigning half of those people to have their drugs replaced by a placebo (Moncrieff 2009).

Any subsequent deterioration in the mental health of those people in the placebo group (the group who have had their medication discontinued) can be interpreted as a return of the 'underlying mental disorder' and therefore taken as evidence that long-term use of psychiatric drugs is necessary to prevent relapse. However, rather than a relapse, it has been suggested that a deterioration in the mental health of those in the placebo group may be a withdrawal or discontinuation effect created by the physiological and psychological stress associated with the cessation of a psychiatric drug (Harrow & Jobe 2013; Healey 2016).

In contrast to the disease-centred model of psychiatric drugs, and the manner in which it can contribute to the subordination of the experiences of people who take those drugs, the drug-centred model is said to imply a more equitable or democratic relationship between mental health professionals and those who use psychiatric drugs (Moncrieff 2008). Understanding psychiatric drugs as powerful psychoactive substances that produce distinctive altered states and a range of cognitive, emotional and physical effects, the drug-centred model places fundamental importance on the subjective experiences of the person using those drugs. Rather than being subordinated to the knowledge and judgements of mental health professionals, it is the subjective experience of the person taking those drugs that is given priority when deciding whether the range of effects that can be produced by a drug are beneficial for the symptoms that comprise an individual's experience of mental distress. Moreover, in contrast to understanding certain drug-induced effects as secondary and tolerable by-products of a drug's supposedly beneficial main effects, the drug-centred model suggests that all of the effects produced by a psychiatric drug should be taken into account when deciding on its effectiveness. In doing so, there is a recognition that while some effects may be experienced by one person as beneficial (such as the manner in which the tranquilising effects of antipsychotics can help some people cope with the positive symptoms of schizophrenia) the same or similar effects might be experienced by another person as unhelpful, undesirable and even disabling.

In contrast with attempts to ensure compliance with a drug-treatment regime that has been predetermined by mental health professionals, the drug-centred model suggests that decisions about whether a psychiatric drug may be helpful is an open, dynamic and collaborative process. That is, whether to use a psychiatric drug as a response to mental distress is an investigation conducted by mental health professionals and the person who may potentially take that drug. In particular, both the person and the practitioner draw upon their respective expertise and experience to explore which drug-induced states and effects may be beneficial. In doing so, there is a recognition of the actual and potential adverse effects of taking a psychiatric drug, both in the short term and the long term, such that the decision about whether a drug is helpful or not becomes an ongoing attempt to balance the actual and potential benefits of a drug against the adverse effects that it may produce. A variety of potential obstacles and challenges can be associated with the establishment of such collaborative, equitable relationships between mental health professionals and those who use mental health services, challenges and opportunities which will be discussed further in Chapter 6. However, such relationships place increased responsibility upon practitioners to not only develop an awareness of the adverse effects of psychiatric drugs, along with a willingness to discuss these with those who use them, but also to develop a more sophisticated understanding of the altered states and subjective experiences that are produced by those drugs.

ACTIVITY 4.2   RESEARCH

Apart from a number of notable exceptions (Gibson *et al.* 2016; Bjornestad *et al.* 2017), there has been a lack of research into service user/survivor experiences of taking psychiatric drugs and which effects people may or may not find helpful. However, such information is increasingly becoming available through, for example, personal written accounts and various forms of electronic media.

For this activity go to John Moore's website and explore the 'Let's Talk Withdrawal' podcast (www.jfmoore.co.uk/podcast.html). There you will not only be able to listen to people's experiences of taking and withdrawing from antidepressants, but you will also find a range of critical perspectives on psychiatric drugs from practitioners, academics and those who use mental health services.

As this activity is based upon your own research, there is no outline answer at the end of the chapter.

By emphasising the importance of the subjective experiences of those taking psychiatric drugs, and the ongoing need to balance the drug-induced effects that a person may find helpful against those effects which they do not, the drug-centred model provides a rationale for what has been referred to as the 'periodic', 'strategic' or 'flexible' use of psychiatric drugs (Moncrieff & Cohen 2009; Healey 2016). That is, there is a recognition that the continuous, long-term use of psychiatric drugs can produce effects that may inhibit, rather than facilitate, the recovery of people who experience mental distress. Therefore, a more effective way to use those drugs may be to employ them when they are needed, such as in response to a deterioration in a person's mental health or to help a person cope with challenging life events. Indeed, there is evidence to suggest that some people already use psychiatric drugs in this flexible or strategic way by increasing, decreasing or omitting doses in response to variations in the symptoms that comprise their experience of mental distress (Deegan & Drake 2006; Britten *et al.* 2010). Therefore, in contrast to the continuous, long-term use of psychiatric drugs, the purpose of the strategic use of those drugs is not simply to alleviate the symptoms associated with mental distress. Rather, in the context of an increased sensitivity to the potentially harmful effects of long-term use of psychiatric drugs, the strategic employment of those drugs attempts to alleviate the symptoms of mental distress while simultaneously seeking to maximise a person's physiological, psychological and social functioning.

ACTIVITY 4.3   RESEARCH

Established by the American psychiatrist Lauren Mosher in 1971, **Soteria** began as an experimental research project that, in response to the emerging dominance of the pharmacological treatment of those newly diagnosed with schizophrenia, investigated the effectiveness of an alternative approach (Mosher *et al.* 2004).

For this activity conduct your own investigations into the Soteria project and provide an overview of its primary concerns. In doing so, attempt to determine the broad aims, methods and results of that project, paying particular attention to the approach that it adopted in relation to the use of psychiatric drugs.

An outline answer is provided at the end of the chapter.

With its emphasis on the flexible and periodic use of psychiatric drugs, the drug-centred model therefore not only recognises the role that those drugs can have in helping people deal with the experiences associated with mental distress, it also highlights their limitations. Rather than being magic bullets that target and correct supposed biological dysfunctions while leaving the rest of the body undisturbed, the drug-centred model maintains that psychiatric drugs are imprecise or blunt instruments. While they can produce effects that some people might find helpful, they also produce short- and long-term effects that others may find unhelpful, unpleasant and even intolerable. As such, there might be some who conclude that the experiences associated with mental distress are less disruptive to their lives than the adverse effects produced by the drugs that are used to treat such distress. In the context of the drug-centred model of psychiatric drugs, such a decision should not be understood as evidence that a person 'lacks insight' or that their mental health is deteriorating, for which more aggressive drug treatment is required. Moreover, it should not simply be assumed that people who experience mental distress do not possess, or are unable to develop, the resilience and strategies to cope without psychiatric drugs (Deegan 2005). Rather, there should be an acknowledgement that alternative non-pharmacological means do exist and practitioners ought to provide the information, support and opportunities for people to explore such means, alongside, or even as an alternative to, the use of psychiatric drugs.

——— PRACTICE ISSUE: PSYCHIATRIC DRUG WITHDRAWAL ———

In response to the use of a psychiatric drug, particularly on a long-term basis, the body will produce a variety of adaptations as it attempts to counteract the effects that the drug has upon a variety of neurotransmitters and brain systems. For example, in response to the manner in which antipsychotics block the action of the neurotransmitter dopamine, the body will increase the number and sensitivity of dopamine receptors in the brain as it adapts to the presence of a drug that is blocking that neurotransmitter. If the drug is stopped, then the body's adaptations will continue to be present and these will give rise to withdrawal symptoms that will persist until the body has returned to normal and the drug-induced adaptations

(Continued)

are no longer present. However, the full range of adaptations that can be induced by the long-term use of psychiatric drugs is not well understood and it may be that some of the body's adaptations persist even after withdrawal (Moncrieff 2008; Breggin 2013).

The experience of withdrawing from a psychiatric drug will be influenced by a number of factors, including the properties of the drug being withdrawn, the rate at which it is withdrawn and the particularities of the person withdrawing. Therefore, the experience of withdrawal can vary among individuals and not everyone who discontinues a psychiatric drug will experience symptoms, while for those who do, the symptoms may not be experienced as problematic. However, it is important to recognise that all psychiatric drugs can produce withdrawal symptoms and these can range from being mild to distressing and even potentially dangerous. Owing to such uncertainties, it is generally recommended that psychiatric drugs should be discontinued in a gradual rather than an abrupt manner (Healey 2016). Wherever possible the decision to withdraw from a psychiatric drug should be an informed, considered decision and it is important that those who decide to do so obtain the necessary information, advice and support about how best to prepare for, and facilitate, the process of psychiatric drug withdrawal.

CHAPTER SUMMARY

This chapter has examined a variety of critical issues surrounding the use of psychiatric drugs and the manner in which they are thought to work. In particular, it has highlighted the way in which ideas about how psychiatric drugs are thought to work are central to a variety of critical debates in contemporary mental health care, including the way in which those drugs are used, the manner in which their potential benefits are balanced against their adverse effects and the extent to which those who use psychiatric drugs are meaningfully involved in decisions about their use. In doing so, we have critically considered the widespread although often implicitly held belief that psychiatric drugs work by targeting and correcting the biological imbalances or dysfunctions that supposedly underlie the emergence and maintenance of mental distress. However, rather than being understood as precise medications or magic bullets that target and correct chemical imbalances, this chapter has also examined an alternative conception of how psychiatric drugs work. This alternative way of thinking about psychiatric drugs suggests that they are powerful psychoactive substances that produce a range of altered states and non-specific physiological and psychological effects. Finally, we have critically considered the implications of these two pharmacological models for how psychiatric drugs are used in mental health care and for the character of the clinical and therapeutic relationship between mental health professionals and those who use psychiatric drugs.

ACTIVITIES: BRIEF OUTLINE ANSWERS

ACTIVITY 4.1 RESEARCH

In conducting your own research into akathisia as an adverse drug reaction you may have discovered that it literally means an 'inability to sit' and is commonly defined in terms of 'restlessness'. Moreover, in attempting to summarise the physiological and psychological experience of akathisia, you may also have found out that it is commonly understood as a subjective sense of 'unease' (and a compulsion to move in order to alleviate this feeling) that is accompanied by a series of observable leg movements, such as a shuffling or swinging of the feet or rocking from one foot to another (Barnes 1989).

While it can be experienced with different levels of intensity, however, defining akathisia in terms of restlessness (both as a subjective sense of unease and a series of observable movements) can minimise the extent of the distress that it can cause. Indeed, it has been suggested that the increased tension, impatience, irritability and impulsivity that can be associated with akathisia means that a more appropriate clinical word for this adverse drug reaction may be **dysphoria**, while a more appropriate everyday description might even be 'mental turmoil' (Healey 2016, p. 31).

ACTIVITY 4.3 RESEARCH

The Soteria project was established in 1971 to investigate whether a minimal medication, relationship-focused approach in a community house was as effective in the treatment of those diagnosed with 'early-episode schizophrenia' as a medication-focused, psychiatric hospital-based approach. The particular therapeutic approach adopted at Soteria was that which Mosher termed 'interpersonal phenomenology' and which focused upon the development of empathic, non-coercive relationships, or 'being-with' the other person. In particular, the experience of mental distress was understood as a potentially meaningful experience that could facilitate personal growth and development (Mosher *et al.* 2004). In comparison with the hospital-based approach, psychiatric drugs were not routinely used at Soteria, and when they were it was at low doses, for short periods of time and in a collaborative, non-coercive manner to alleviate distress that was not responding to interpersonal phenomenology.

Although the project ended in 1983, owing to 'administrative problems' and a lack of funding, the Soteria approach was found to be at least as effective as a hospital-based approach for the treatment of early-episode schizophrenia at both the six-week and two-year follow-up periods – results that were achieved with minimal use of psychiatric drugs and therefore with the reduced risk of adverse drug reactions (Mosher *et al.* 1995; Bola & Mosher 2003). It has been suggested that the Soteria project remains an experimental approach that requires further research to determine its therapeutic effects. However, investigations into a number of projects that have adopted 'the Soteria paradigm' as a response to early-episode schizophrenia have similarly shown that it is at least as effective, and in some instances superior, to a medication-focused and hospital-based approach (Calton *et al.* 2008).

FURTHER READING

- **Healey D** (2016) *Psychiatric Drugs Explained*, 6th edition. London: Elsevier.

This book is an established guide to the use of psychiatric drugs in the management of various forms of mental distress that provides an accessible and comprehensive account of the potentially beneficial and adverse effects associated with their use.

- Kirsch I (2009) *The Emperor's New Drugs: Exploding the Antidepressant Myth*. London: The Bodley Head.

A stimulating investigation into the published and unpublished data from clinical trials on antidepressants in order to maintain that, rather than correcting a chemical imbalance, most (if not all) of the perceived benefits of antidepressants are due to the placebo effect.

- Moncrieff J (2008) *The Myth of the Chemical Cure: A Critique of Psychiatric Drug Treatment*. Basingstoke: Palgrave Macmillan.

A sustained critical account of the disease-centred and drug-centred models of psychiatric medication, along with a discussion of the implications of those models for people who use, and work within, contemporary mental health services.

- Whitaker R (2015) *Anatomy of an Epidemic: Magic Bullets, Psychiatric Drugs, and the Astonishing Rise of Mental Illness in America*. New York, NY: Broadway Books.

A wide-ranging and provocative book which proposes that, rather than being an effective treatment for mental distress, the increasingly widespread and long-term use of psychiatric drugs has contributed to an increased incidence of mental distress.

USEFUL WEBSITES

- www.comingoff.com

This is the website for Coming Off Psychiatric Medication, established by both mental health professionals and those who have taken psychiatric drugs, which provides information, advice and support about the psychiatric drug withdrawal process.

- www.soterianetwork.org.uk

Here you will find the website for the Soteria Network, which engages in a variety of activities to promote the development of psychiatric drug-free and minimum medication environments for people experiencing psychosis.

5

PSYCHOLOGICAL THERAPIES

CHAPTER AIMS

By the end of this chapter you will be able to:

* appraise the effectiveness of psychological therapies;
* debate the individualistic focus of psychological therapies;
* assess community psychology as an alternative to psychological therapies.

INTRODUCTION

👥 CASE STUDY

Clara is a 24-year-old single mother with two young children who began to have a range of distressing physical and psychological experiences just over six months ago. Following an assessment by her general practitioner it was suggested to Clara that she might be experiencing 'generalised anxiety disorder' for which she was prescribed, and has been taking, psychiatric medication. Although she thinks that the medication has helped alleviate some of her distressing experiences, Clara did not feel that the origin of those experiences was being explored or addressed. She was therefore offered the opportunity to see a 'therapist' and, although Clara has so far only had two therapy sessions, she is finding it to be a positive experience. While the therapist has introduced Clara to various psychological strategies, she has valued the opportunity to discuss her experiences and current difficulties. As a consequence of doing so, Clara has felt less isolated with those difficulties and now feels that her experiences, rather than being minimised, are being acknowledged and validated.

The use of psychological interventions as a response to mental distress has become an established part of contemporary mental health care and, as illustrated in the above case study, those who use mental health services commonly express a preference for them over other forms of intervention such as psychiatric drugs

(McHugh *et al.* 2013). Partly as a response to this, there has been a commitment to improve access to a range of psychological therapies and, while once the province of trained psychotherapists and counsellors, practitioners from a variety of disciplines are increasingly incorporating counselling and psychotherapeutic techniques into their everyday practice. Despite the expressed preference for psychological interventions among those with experience of mental distress, and the increasing use of psychotherapeutic techniques among diverse groups of health care professionals, a variety of critical issues surround this form of intervention (Masson 1988; Furedi 2004; Proctor 2017). For example, there are critical examinations of the manner in which psychological therapies are used in the clinical setting and challenging considerations about trust, the imbalance of power and various forms of potential exploitation. There are also complex critical discussions about the quality of research into the effectiveness of psychological interventions and the appropriateness of the methods used to investigate that effectiveness. In addition, there are a variety of sociological, political and philosophical critiques of psychotherapy which reflect critically upon the supposed expansion of a 'therapeutic, confessional culture' into widening areas of people's lives and what were traditionally thought of as non-therapeutic domains such as schools, universities and the workplace.

The purpose of this chapter is therefore to introduce you to a variety of critical issues surrounding the use of psychological therapies in contemporary mental health care. While a diversity of such interventions are used to respond to mental distress, the chapter will begin by considering their effectiveness and whether they produce beneficial outcomes for those who receive and engage with them. In the context of the dominance of some forms of psychological intervention, we shall then consider if any one specific form of therapy is more effective than any other, as well as the way in which the quality of the therapeutic relationship, and the variety of relational factors that comprise that relationship, can influence this effectiveness. Moreover, despite the diverse range of available psychological therapies, many of them can be understood as possessing an individualistic orientation in so far they seek to facilitate change 'within' the individual. This chapter will therefore move on to discuss the social and political implications of understanding and responding to mental distress in terms of this individualistic orientation and, in particular, its potential

Table 5.1 Psychological interventions

Psychodynamic approaches	Humanistic-existential approaches	Cognitive-behavioural approaches	Integrative-eclectic approaches
Freudian psychoanalysis Jungian analytical psychology Kleinian analysis Lacanian psychoanalysis	Person-centred therapy Transactional analysis Gestalt therapy Existential therapy Reality therapy Logotherapy Narrative therapy	Behaviour therapy Cognitive therapy Rational emotive behaviour therapy Dialectical behaviour therapy Acceptance and commitment therapy	Multimodal therapy Cognitive analytic therapy Transtheoretical model Skilled helper model Solution-focused brief therapy

limitations. Finally, in contrast to the individualistic focus of various psychological therapies, we shall examine a variety of emerging initiatives, both within and beyond the mental health system, that can be understood as being consistent with the field of practice that is known as community psychology. In particular, we shall consider the way in which community psychology interventions can be employed to understand and respond to the manner in which a variety of social and material conditions can contribute to the emergence and maintenance of mental distress.

ACTIVITY 5.1   TEAM WORKING

A diverse range of psychological interventions are used in contemporary mental health care and it can be a challenge making sense of that diversity. A common approach, as shown in Table 5.1, is to think of particular interventions as having certain theoretical and therapeutic similarities and belonging to specific 'schools'.

Despite similarities between psychological interventions, it is important to recognise that there are also considerable differences. While it can help to comprehend the range of available psychotherapies, such categorisation should be understood as provisional and open to discussion, dispute and revision.

For this activity choose one psychological intervention from either the psychodynamic, humanistic-existential, cognitive-behavioural or integrative-eclectic schools. In doing so, conduct your own research into the principles and practices associated with that intervention and share your findings with your colleagues.

As this activity is based upon your own research, there is no outline answer at the end of the chapter.

THE EFFECTIVENESS OF PSYCHOLOGICAL THERAPIES

One of the most important and enduring critical questions surrounding the use of psychological interventions, especially in the context of evidence-based practice within contemporary mental health care, concerns their effectiveness and whether they produce beneficial outcomes for those who receive them. Despite its apparent simplicity, such a question is a particularly challenging one in so far as it involves a variety of complex practical, theoretical and methodological considerations (Comer & Kendall 2013; Ogles 2013). Such considerations involve, for example, clarifying what is meant by a beneficial, positive or successful outcome. The question also necessitates an examination of whether any apparent benefits are a result of the psychological intervention being used, as opposed to a variety of other 'extra-therapeutic factors', such as the passage of time, the occurrence of fortuitous events or the favourable expectations of those receiving therapy. In addition, it involves a consideration of whether the research methods used to evaluate the effectiveness of a particular psychological therapy are appropriate for the area under investigation. However, when such complexities are taken into account (and whether the concern is with the outcomes of psychological therapies in general terms or the effects of particular interventions for specific forms of mental distress), it has been suggested that the evidence from thousands of research studies that have been conducted since the 1950s indicates that psychological therapies (with a number of important caveats) do produce a beneficial effect upon the well-being of those who receive them (Cooper 2008; Wampold & Imel 2015).

In particular, when compared with those individuals who do not receive a psychological intervention, or who receive a 'placebo psychological intervention' (understood as some form of non-specific, listening-based befriending), the evidence suggests that those who receive a genuine therapy based on recognised psychological principles experience positive, clinically significant effects on their levels of mental distress. Moreover, the research indicates that these beneficial outcomes are not due to extra-therapeutic factors such as the passage of time, the occurrence of fortuitous events or the favourable expectations of those receiving a psychological intervention (Lambert 2013). However, when considering the effectiveness of psychological therapies, it is important to recognise a distinction that is made between their efficacy and their effectiveness. While the former refers to the outcomes that psychological therapies produce under strictly controlled experimental conditions (as in **randomised controlled trials**), the latter refers to the outcomes that psychological therapies produce in the context of 'routine, real-world' therapeutic practice. The majority of studies into the outcomes of psychological interventions have been conducted under strict experimental conditions with highly selected participants, and have therefore assessed the efficacy of those interventions. However, the available research indicates that psychological therapies are also effective in so far as they have been found to produce beneficial, clinically significant outcomes when assessed in the context of routine therapeutic practice with people who have multiple, diverse and complex psychological problems (Stiles *et al.* 2008; Lambert 2013).

 CASE STUDY

Anisha has been a qualified mental health professional for almost 18 months and during that time she has started to incorporate various psychotherapeutic techniques into her practice. While her own reflections and clinical experiences have led her to believe that such techniques are beneficial, she has recently discovered that the available research also provides evidence for the efficacy and effectiveness of psychological interventions. Moreover, she has not only found out that service users/survivors express a general preference for psychological therapies over other forms of intervention but, somewhat to her surprise, that those interventions may be at least as efficacious as psychiatric drugs for some forms of mental distress. Such research findings, along with her own reflections and experiences, have led her to consider developing her ability to deliver psychological interventions. Following a brief investigation, however, she has discovered that a wide range of psychotherapies are now available. As she investigates further, she is becoming increasingly confused about which might be the best to pursue in order to develop her ability to productively respond to mental distress.

While recognising that psychological interventions can produce beneficial outcomes for those who experience mental distress, you may, like Anisha in the above case study, be uncertain about which is the most beneficial. It has repeatedly been asserted, however, that when different psychotherapeutic approaches are compared with one another, the evidence indicates that there are minimal differences between them in terms of the beneficial effects that they produce. Indeed, where different approaches have been found to produce different outcomes, it has been suggested that those differences are so small that, at least for research purposes, they ought to be considered as 'negligible' and 'non-significant' (Smith & Glass 1977; Luborsky et al. 2002; Wampold & Imel 2015). Given the manner in which certain psychological interventions, most notably cognitive behavioural therapy, have achieved prominence in contemporary mental health care, the claim that different psychotherapeutic approaches do not produce significantly different outcomes may seem somewhat surprising. However, when different therapies are assessed under strict experimental conditions, and when they are assessed in the real-world context of routine therapeutic practice, there is a substantial body of evidence to indicate that there is minimal difference in the efficacy and the effectiveness of one psychological intervention over any other. As Cooper (2008) has concluded in summarising this evidence, 'it would appear that most therapies seem to be effective with most things they have been tested for, with little evidence that any one approach is much more effective than any other' (p. 52).

The finding that different psychotherapeutic approaches produce roughly the same beneficial outcomes – a finding which has come to be known as the **dodo bird verdict** (Rosenzweig 1936; Luborsky et al. 1975) – is one of the most well-established in the field of psychotherapy research and various explanations for it have been proposed. For example, it has been suggested that different psychotherapies might actually produce significantly different outcomes, but, historically, these may not have been detected by existing research methods (Lambert 2013). However, one of the most prominent explanations for the dodo bird verdict is that, despite their individual differences, most psychotherapies share certain elements or factors and it is the presence of these common factors that leads different therapies to produce roughly equivalent outcomes. It is these factors that can be common to all psychotherapies that are therefore thought to be the most important elements for producing beneficial outcomes rather than the specific techniques that are unique to particular approaches (such as the identification of 'negative thoughts' in cognitive behavioural therapy or interpretations in psychoanalysis that connect present mental distress to past relationships). While a variety of these non-specific, common factors have been found to be significant in producing beneficial outcomes across all psychotherapies (such as the presence of social support and fortuitous events), the most important is said to be the quality of the therapeutic relationship between the 'therapist' and the 'client' and the relational factors which form that relationship (Duncan et al. 2010; Norcross 2011; Goldsmith et al. 2015).

——— PRACTICE ISSUE: THERAPEUTIC RELATIONAL FACTORS ———

In developing therapeutic relationships with those experiencing mental distress, the variety of factors which form that relationship can be intimately bound to one another and deeply embedded in the interpersonal character of the therapeutic encounter. For research purposes, it can therefore be a particular challenge to isolate those factors and discover their particular effects. Despite this, there is evidence to suggest that a number of relational factors have a positive, clinically significant effect upon the well-being of those who receive psychological interventions (Cooper 2008; Wampold 2015). These relational factors include:

- positive regard or the ability of the therapist to maintain an acceptance of, and non-possessive warmth towards, the client;
- an agreement between the client and the therapist about the goals of the psychological intervention and a collaborative pursuit of these goals;
- the provision of feedback to clients that includes evaluations of, and appropriate emotional responses to, various behaviours;
- genuineness or congruence in which the therapist is able to communicate sensitively their experiences during the course of the therapeutic encounter;
- empathy or the ability to have an engaged understanding of the client's experience and to display this understanding to those receiving therapy;
- the management of countertransference, where this is understood as the therapist's reactions to the client that are based upon the therapist's needs, values and 'unresolved conflicts';
- skilful self-disclosure or the ability of the therapist to provide appropriate personal information during the course of therapy;
- the ability of the therapist to repair and resolve tensions, ruptures or breakdowns in the therapeutic relationship.

The research evidence in favour of the finding that different psychotherapeutic approaches produce roughly equivalent outcomes because of the therapeutic relationship and other non-specific factors is a matter of ongoing debate and dispute (Hunsley & Di Giulio 2002; Westmacott & Hunsley 2007; Marcus *et al.* 2014). For example, it has been suggested that the contemporary evidence indicates that some forms of psychotherapy do produce more beneficial and clinically significant outcomes than others, with particular emphasis placed on the efficacy of cognitive behavioural therapy for certain forms of mental distress – such as bulimia nervosa, anxiety disorders and the management of anger, aggression and 'general stress' (Hofmann *et al.* 2012). However, it has been argued that the research to establish the apparent therapeutic superiority of one psychological intervention over another can be compromised by a variety of methodological problems. One of the most significant, for example, is the researcher allegiance effect, in which researchers will inadvertently influence the research in ways that support the psychotherapeutic approach that they favour or to which they have an allegiance (Munder *et al.* 2013; Dragioti *et al.* 2015). Indeed, in contrast to the supposed superiority of cognitive behavioural therapy, it has not only been suggested that it is no more effective than any other psychotherapeutic approach (Barth *et al.* 2013; Cuijpers *et al.* 2013), but that it may even be producing less beneficial outcomes than it did in the past, particularly as a treatment for depression (Johnsen & Friborg 2015).

Partly as a consequence of the seeming intractability of such debates, there have been calls to move beyond the attempt to discover whether it is non-specific common factors that produce beneficial outcomes in psychotherapy, or whether such outcomes are the result of particular psychological techniques associated with certain psychotherapeutic approaches. That is, rather than seeking to conclusively determine if it is the therapeutic relationship or specific therapeutic techniques that produce beneficial outcomes, it is more productive to begin from the assumption that the therapeutic encounter is a complex phenomenon in which a variety of approaches, techniques and relational qualities all have the potential to facilitate psychological well-being (Castonguay & Beutler 2006; Cooper & McLeod 2011). Indeed, it is important to recognise that in your 'everyday' mental health practice, the particular counselling skills and psychotherapeutic techniques that you might employ will be intimately bound to the particular manner in which you relate to those who use mental health services. Therefore, while you may – like Anisha in the above case study – be keen to develop specific psychotherapeutic techniques and integrate them into your mental health practice, the research into the effect of relational factors on therapeutic outcomes suggests that at least equal consideration should be given to developing an ability to establish and maintain collaborative, therapeutic alliances with those who experience mental distress as is given to the development and implementation of particular psychotherapeutic techniques.

ACTIVITY 5.2   TEAM WORKING

The therapeutic encounter is a complex and dynamic phenomenon in which a variety of factors can have a beneficial effect upon the well-being of those who receive psychological interventions. As well as the therapeutic relationship and psychotherapeutic techniques, the client's expectations that the intervention will work and extra-therapeutic events (such as spontaneous remission, self-change, social support and fortuitous events) have also been identified as having a positive influence. Moreover, not only is there evidence to suggest that these various elements are clinically significant, but research also exists to indicate the relative effect, in percentage terms, that each of these elements has upon the outcomes associated with psychological therapies (Norcross & Lambert 2011).

For this activity discuss with your colleagues how much effect you think the following four elements have upon successful psychotherapeutic change. As you do so, attempt to reach a consensus about how much effect, in percentage terms, is attributable to:

- psychotherapeutic techniques;
- the client's favourable expectations;
- extra-therapeutic events;
- the therapeutic relationship.

An outline answer is provided at the end of the chapter.

While many people who receive psychological interventions experience a beneficial effect, it is important to recognise that not only do some people receive no benefit but they can also experience negative effects as a result of those interventions (Bowie *et al.* 2016; Crawford *et al.* 2016). Although there has been minimal research into the harmful effects of psychological therapies, it has been claimed that approximately 5 to 10 per cent of those receiving a psychological intervention for mental distress experience a deterioration in their symptoms, while this rises to approximately 7 to 15 per cent for those receiving psychotherapy for substance use problems (Moos 2005; Lilienfeld 2007). However, the full extent to which people may be harmed by psychological therapies remains unclear and a variety of reasons for this have been proposed (Nutt & Sharpe 2008; Dimidjian & Hollon 2010; Vaughan *et al.* 2014). For example, there is a lack of agreement about what constitutes a negative effect or adverse treatment reaction in psychotherapy, such that, in all but the most clear cases, there are methodological and clinical challenges in deciding what is a negative outcome. It has also been suggested that there exists an enduring assumption among researchers, therapists and the wider public that psychological interventions, as opposed to psychiatric drugs, are unlikely to cause harm because they are based around talking. Moreover, it has been claimed that research trials into the efficacy of psychological interventions, especially in comparison to research trials into psychiatric drugs, fail to adequately monitor and report the presence of potential or actual harms, negative effects and adverse treatment reactions.

While considerable effort has been made to investigate how psychological interventions may produce beneficial outcomes, it has been suggested that a similar degree of effort needs to be made to consider how those interventions might have negative effects upon a person's mental distress and well-being (Berk & Parker 2009; Barlow 2010; Scott & Young 2016). Not only does there need to be greater clarification for both research and clinical purposes about what constitutes harm in psychotherapy, the processes by which harm occurs and what specific techniques may be more likely to cause harm than others, there also needs to be a recognition that psychological therapies may have a variety of broader detrimental effects upon an individual's life. For example, as well as measuring psychotherapeutic harm in terms of a deterioration in the symptoms associated with a particular manifestation of mental distress, it has been suggested that a variety of other effects ought to be included in a comprehensive assessment of the harms that psychological interventions may produce (Lilienfeld 2007; Linden & Schermuly-Haupt 2014; Parry *et al.* 2016). These should include the emergence of new symptoms or a person's increased concern about existing symptoms during the course of the therapeutic encounter; an assessment of whether a person is becoming dependent upon the therapist or feeling humiliated, intimidated or manipulated by them; and a recognition of the potential of psychological interventions to produce a wide range of adverse effects upon an individual's personal relationships, occupation and general quality of life.

CONCEPT SUMMARY: THERAPY CULTURE

While it has been suggested that there is a need for more research into the harms that psychological interventions can produce, there have been sociological and political critiques of the emergence of what has been termed 'therapy culture' (Furedi 2004; Ecclestone & Hayes 2009). Therapy culture refers to the manner in which there is said to have been an expansion of psychotherapeutic concepts, terminology and practices throughout contemporary Western societies and into what were traditionally thought of as non-therapeutic domains, such as schools, universities and the workplace. As a result, there is a tendency for people to begin to understand their experiences, their identity and increasing areas of their life in psychotherapeutic terms, such that events which were previously regarded as normal, albeit unpleasant aspects of human existence (e.g. sadness, worry and frustration) become reformulated as potential threats to psychological well-being.

As a consequence of the emergence and expansion of a therapy culture, it has been proposed that people increasingly think of themselves as emotionally vulnerable and as possessing a 'fragile self'. In doing so, the variety of potentially challenging events that comprise the course of people's lives begin to be reformulated as experiences which can not only cause psychological distress, but which may also require psychotherapeutic treatment and the intervention of mental health professionals to manage. Therefore, while psychological therapies are often presented as being concerned with facilitating a person's self-awareness, self-discovery and even self-realisation, Furedi (2004) has argued that 'the therapeutic imperative is not so much towards the realisation of self-fulfilment as the promotion of self-limitation. It posits the self in distinctly fragile and feeble form and insists that the management of life requires the continuous intervention of therapeutic expertise' (p. 21).

THE LIMITATIONS OF PSYCHOLOGICAL THERAPIES

👤👤👤 CASE STUDY

Vasile is a 33-year-old married man with two young children who has been referred to Keira, a mental health professional, experiencing features associated with a diagnosis of depression. During his initial meeting with Keira, Vasile attributed these experiences to the loss of his job 12 months ago following what his employer referred to as 'efficiency savings'. Although he found new employment six months later, Vasile has described it as 'low paid, insecure work' that has made his existing financial problems worse and has created increased tensions with his wife. As a consequence, Vasile has suggested that he is beginning to feel 'worthless', that he ought to have found a better job by now and that by being unable to do so his wife and children are beginning to think of him as a 'failure'.

Having reflected upon Vasile's difficulties with a colleague, and noting how he is expressing a variety of 'negative thoughts' about himself and his situation, Keira has concluded that a

(Continued)

short period of low-intensity cognitive behavioural therapy might be a productive response to his distress. Although Vasile has no understanding of this intervention, he is keen to accept any form of assistance and he has agreed to one session a week for the next six weeks. Having received training in cognitive behavioural therapy, Keira has therefore decided to deliver that psychological intervention herself. In doing so, she has devised a provisional account of the manner in which Vasile's mental distress may have developed and how his own thoughts or 'cognitive processes' might be maintaining that distress.

In addition to their efficacy and effectiveness, a variety of critical considerations surround the theoretical and therapeutic focus of psychological interventions, and, in particular, the social and political implications of that focus. To begin to understand these critical concerns, it is productive to recognise that, despite their diverse theoretical principles and therapeutic practices, many psychological therapies possess an individualistic orientation in so far as they are concerned with facilitating change within the individual and, variously, with the individual's thoughts, feelings and behaviours (Richardson & Zeddies 2001; Orford 2008). While a multiplicity of reasons for this predominately individualistic focus have been given, it is commonly said to be a result of the enduring assumption (an assumption shared with the biomedical model of mental distress) that the origin or cause of mental distress is to be understood as primarily located within the individual (Prilleltensky 1994; Smail 2011). In contrast with the biomedical model, however, the cause of mental distress is not to be understood as a consequence of some form of biological dysfunction or chemical imbalance. Rather, by adopting the biomedical model's language or **discourse of deficit**, various psychological therapies are said to either explicitly or implicitly attribute mental distress to some form of 'psychological dysfunction' such as 'neurotic development' and 'ego weakness' in psychoanalysis, or, more recently, 'faulty cognitions' and 'thinking errors' in cognitive behavioural therapy (Gergen 1990; Boyle 2015; Coles *et al.* 2015).

However, while mental distress finds its expression within or through the individual, the emergence and the maintenance of that distress can be understood as having its origins 'outside' or 'beyond' the individual. As highlighted in Chapter 2, a range of social, economic and political factors – or what are commonly referred to as social determinants – can profoundly influence the everyday, material conditions of people's lives and, in doing so, increase the possibility of the occurrence of mental distress throughout the course of those lives (Compton & Shim 2015). These can include those proximal social determinants that have a 'close proximity' to an individual and which can thereby influence a person's mental health from a comparatively 'short distance' and in a direct and immediate way. Such proximal social determinants include unemployment or low-paid, insecure employment; poor housing, insecure living conditions and homelessness; and low-quality neighbourhoods with multiple social stressors such as vandalism, noise pollution and crime. In contrast, a number of distal social determinants that exist 'farther away' from an individual can exert their influence upon a person's mental health, and they do so from a 'greater distance' and often in an indirect way through other mediating factors. Such distal social determinants include local and national decisions on health and welfare expenditure, the availability of affordable housing, policing levels and migration policies, as well as the occurrence of economic recessions and the levels of wealth inequality throughout society.

CONCEPT SUMMARY: THE POWER HORIZON

Introduced by the psychologist and psychotherapist David Smail (2014), the power horizon is a productive spatial metaphor that can help us to understand why many psychological interventions (and explanations of mental distress in general) primarily locate the origin of that distress within the individual rather than being associated with the range of social factors that can affect people's lives. In doing so, the power horizon refers to the field of social factors or 'powers' within which each person exists and suggests that those powers influence the individual from varying degrees of distance. In particular, it proposes that some of the most influential social powers (such as economic recessions, governmental policies and the mass media) exist at such a distance from an individual that they are often 'beyond the horizon' of our everyday perception and comprehension.

If such distant social powers are perceived at all, then their influence is thought to be so 'vague and diffuse' that they are treated as being largely irrelevant for a useful understanding and practical response to mental distress (Smail 2014, p. 32). Therefore, when the influence of social powers upon mental distress is recognised, attention is often given to those which exist 'closer to us' and 'within the horizon' of our everyday perception and comprehension. Accordingly, while the influence of family dynamics and interpersonal relations has been the focus of some psychological therapies, most attention has been given to those powers or factors that are perceived as having the greatest proximity to a person and of being the most receptive to psychotherapeutic intervention: namely, the thoughts, feelings and behaviour of the individual.

It has been suggested that mental distress is a multifaceted and multilevel phenomenon such that the attempt to understand that distress, and the variety of factors which can potentially contribute to its emergence and maintenance, is often 'staggeringly complex' (Kendler 2005, p. 439). Indeed, rather than simply being attributable to one factor, it has been proposed that mental distress is perhaps most productively understood as a consequence of processes that act at the micro and macro level both within and outside of the individual, processes that are best understood from a combination of sociological, psychological and biological perspectives (Kendler 2008). However, while practitioners are said to have a tendency to favour approaches that attribute mental distress to some form of quality or characteristic within the individual, those who use mental health services are more likely to provide social and material explanations for their experience of distress

(Bostock *et al.* 2012; Beresford *et al.* 2016). In the above case study, for example, Vasile appears to understand his mental distress in terms of a variety of interdependent proximal and distal social determinants which are significantly influencing the material conditions of his everyday existence. In particular, he seems to attribute his distress to the loss of his job 12 months ago and only being able to find new employment that he describes as low paid and insecure. In addition, he also suggests that these social factors are making his existing financial problems worse, creating increased tensions with his wife and having a detrimental effect upon his self-esteem and feelings of self-worth.

Although Vasile appears to provide a social and material explanation for his mental distress, Keira has chosen to understand and respond to his current difficulties by using a cognitive behavioural approach which locates the origin and the maintenance of mental distress within the individual. It is important to recognise, however, that cognitive behavioural therapy is not a single, unified and static psychological intervention. Rather, it is a diverse and evolving family of therapeutic approaches and it is therefore necessary to be cautious when making general assertions about the principles and practices associated with these approaches. Despite this diversity, however, a central assumption shared by the variety of cognitive behavioural approaches is that the social factors and events to which an individual may be subject are not, in and of themselves, the origin of mental distress. Instead, the fundamental theoretical principle of any cognitive behavioural approach is that the source of such distress is to be attributed to the individual's thoughts, beliefs or interpretations of the social factors and events to which they may be subject (Kennerley *et al.* 2016). Indeed, in articulating the fundamental theoretical assumption and philosophical orientation of this psychotherapeutic approach, both Aaron Beck (1979) and Albert Ellis (1962) – arguably the two most influential figures in the development of modern cognitive behavioural therapy – proposed that these can be understood as being encapsulated in the famous declaration of the ancient Stoic philosopher Epictetus (2008) that 'It is not events that disturb people, it is their judgements concerning them' (p. 223).

ACTIVITY 5.3   REFLECTION

In their subsequent meetings, Keira has presented her cognitive behavioural account of the origin of Vasile's mental distress and the way in which his own cognitive processes may be maintaining that distress (such as the thought that he is 'worthless' and that his wife and children think of him as a 'failure'). She has also encouraged Vasile to keep a diary to begin to recognise these and other similar 'negative automatic thoughts', to record the situations in which they occur and to note the physical sensations, emotions and behaviours that are associated with them. In addition, Keira has started to help Vasile examine and reconsider the evidence for these 'unproductive cognitions' and to replace them with more 'objective, balanced and productive thoughts'.

For this activity reflect upon Vasile's situation in the above case study and the variety of social determinants and psychological factors that may have contributed to the emergence and maintenance of his mental distress. As you do so, attempt to identify what a cognitive behavioural approach might be able to achieve in this situation and also consider critically what might be the limitations of that approach.
An outline answer is provided at the end of the chapter.

The manner in which various psychological therapies possess a predominately individualistic orientation, and maintain theoretical assumptions that locate the origin of mental distress primarily within the individual, can be understood as having significant social and political implications. In particular, by understanding mental distress in such individualistic terms, and inviting those who receive psychological interventions to understand their distress in this way, those interventions are said to be characterised by a tendency to obscure, mystify and even neglect the social context within which people's lives are lived (Smail 2011). Indeed, it has been suggested that the terminology or language which is associated with psychological therapies, and the language which characterises mental health care more generally, serves to obscure an understanding of the challenging social context within which people's lives can be lived and the way in which that context can contribute to mental distress. In particular, there is said to be a notable absence of crucial and critical social concepts such as injustice, inequality and discrimination in favour of the individualistic and largely decontextualised language associated with individual dysfunctions, disorders and deficits (Boyle 2011). It has even been suggested that the term 'mental' or 'psychological distress' is a misnomer in so far as it 'dislocates and disembodies distress', divorcing it from the variety of social factors and material conditions that can contribute to its emergence, and instead shifts the focus onto the individual and their mental or psychological processes (Smail 2014, p. 23).

By obscuring an appreciation of the range of social factors and material conditions that can contribute to mental distress, it has been suggested that psychological therapies can serve a variety of political, ideological and economic interests. That is, by locating the origin of mental distress primarily within the individual and their psychological processes, political attention and resources can be directed to the provision of brief, short-term and relatively inexpensive psychological interventions rather than the more financially and politically demanding task of attempting to address the multiple challenges that can characterise the social context within which people's lives are lived. As Epstein (1995) has suggested, 'This is an immensely attractive strategy for a society that is reluctant to allocate substantial funds to address its problems', as well as being consistent with any political ideology 'that is unwilling to accept broad-based social expenditures to provide greater social equality through government action' (p. 6). Indeed, it has been suggested that the individualistic orientation associated with various psychological therapies has in this way become consistent with the interests of contemporary capitalist society, and, in particular, the economic and political ideology referred to as neoliberalism (Ferraro 2016). Thus, those therapies are said to effectively divert attention away from the need for state intervention and public expenditure to address injustice, inequality and discrimination, and instead shift the focus onto accommodating individuals to unjust, oppressive and damaging social, material and environmental conditions (Moloney 2013).

To maintain that a political consequence of the individualistic orientation of many psychological interventions is to divert attention away from the need to address the multiple social challenges which can contribute to mental distress, is not to suggest that those who provide such interventions actively endorse the political, ideological and economic interests that such an orientation can serve. Rather, this individualistic focus can be understood as primarily emerging from, and being maintained by, a variety of pragmatic considerations. As highlighted above within the context of the power horizon, the way in which a multiplicity of distal and proximal social determinants can contribute to mental distress may appear so vague and diffuse, and the possibility of improving the social and material conditions of people's lives can appear so complex and beyond the scope of everyday mental health practice, that individual explanations and responses to mental distress can appear seductively simple. That is, confronted with the theoretical complexity and practical challenges associated with a social and material understanding of mental distress, the individualistic orientation of various psychological therapies can provide mental health professionals with an accessible account of what contributes to the emergence and maintenance of that distress. Moreover, those psychological approaches also offer the alluring possibility of developing a set of practical skills and techniques to respond to such distress that, with relatively minimal training and allocation of resources, can readily be implemented by any individual practitioner.

ALTERNATIVES TO PSYCHOLOGICAL THERAPIES

 CASE STUDY

Having incorporated a variety of counselling skills and psychotherapeutic techniques into his mental health practice, Anthony has recently been introduced to critiques concerning their individualistic focus. As a result, he has been reflecting upon how those interventions, by seeking to facilitate change within the individual, may obscure or neglect the way in which various social and material factors can contribute to mental distress. While Anthony maintains that psychological interventions, and cognitive behavioural approaches in particular, are a productive way to understand and respond to mental distress, he is beginning to develop a greater appreciation of how the challenging social context in which people's lives are lived can contribute to the experience of such distress. However, although he recognises that a comprehensive response to mental distress ought to include strategies designed to address this context, he thinks that the work necessary to improve the social and material conditions of people's lives is so formidable that he cannot see what individual practitioners, and even existing mental health services, could realistically do to support such initiatives.

The critique of the individualistic orientation of psychological therapies, and the suggestion that this orientation can divert attention away from the multiple social challenges which can contribute to mental distress, should not be understood as a rejection of the significant contribution that these interventions can make. As high-lighted at the beginning of this chapter, not only do those who use mental health services commonly express a preference for psychological therapies over other forms of intervention (such as psychiatric drugs), but the available research suggests that such therapies produce, in the main, a beneficial and clinically significant effect upon the levels of mental distress and well-being of those who receive them. Therefore, rather than a rejection of the contribution that psychological interventions can make to contemporary mental health care, the critique of their predominately individual-istic focus should be understood as seeking to foster a critical appraisal of both their strengths and limitations. As a consequence of such an appraisal, a comprehensive theoretical and therapeutic approach to mental distress, while acknowledging the efficacy and effectiveness of psychological therapies, ought to give at least equal consideration to an understanding of how the social and material conditions of people's lives can contribute to mental distress. In addition, it has been suggested that such an appraisal should lead to the development and implementation of effec-tive local, national and international strategies designed to address those contributory factors (Allen *et al.* 2014; Compton & Shim 2015).

While they have traditionally dominated mental health care, the individualistic interventions implemented by mental health professionals (such as psychological therapy, psychiatric medication and mental health education) are said to have, at best, a minimal effect upon the multiple challenges which can characterise the social context in which people's lives are lived (Shim *et al.* 2014). However, like Anthony in the above case study, you may feel that the work necessary to address the various social determinants that can contribute to mental distress (such as poor employ-ment, homelessness and poverty) is largely beyond the scope of individual mental health professionals, and even wider mental health services. Indeed, it has been proposed that in addition to the individual interventions of practitioners, what is required are progressive social, economic and political policies that are focused upon creating environments, communities and whole societies that are more con-ducive to people's psychological well-being (Clements & Davies 2013; Kinderman 2014). In response, mental health professionals are said to have a role to play by actively participating in various political activities to advocate for such progressive policies. However, the development and implementation of the structural reforms needed to address the various complex and challenging social determinants that can contribute to mental distress require concerted political will and action, and this, it has been proposed, cannot primarily be a matter for individual practitioners but must ultimately be a matter for government (Smail 2014).

ACTIVITY 5.4   RESEARCH

In *Social Determinants of Mental Health* the WHO (2014) investigate the range of social factors which can contribute to mental distress. In doing so, they not only propose that the actions needed to address those conditions require the participation of mental health services at the individual and community levels, but they also demand initiatives at the structural level by social institutions, governments and international organisations.

For this activity access and reflect upon the WHO's document (www.who.int/mental_health/publications/gulbenkian_paper_social_determinants_of_mental_health/en/). As you do so, consider the complex, multi-layered and multi-sectoral strategies that are considered necessary to address the social determinants that can contribute to the emergence and maintenance of mental distress.

As this activity is based upon your own research, there is no outline answer at the end of the chapter.

While recognising the need to advocate for progressive social, economic and political policies that foster psychological well-being, there are a number of emerging movements and initiatives, both within and beyond the mental health system, that seek to address directly the social and material factors that can contribute to mental distress. Although such movements are diverse, have varying objectives and are conducted by a multiplicity of professional and non-professional groups, they can be understood as sharing many of the principles and concerns that are consistent with the field of practice that is known as community psychology. As a sub-discipline of psychology, community psychology has a complex, varied and rich theoretical and therapeutic history, and has developed at different rates in different countries. The reasons for this are multifaceted but it can be understood, in part, as a result of the diverse social, economic and political objectives that community psychology approaches have sought to achieve in the different contexts within which they have emerged and been implemented (Reich *et al.* 2007; Walker *et al.* 2012). Community psychology can therefore be a particular challenge to define concisely, not least because, in seeking to achieve a range of objectives, it shares many theoretical and practical concerns with a variety of other disciplines and areas of knowledge, such as public health, community development, anthropology, sociology, social work and political science (Kloos *et al.* 2012).

Despite the challenge of providing a concise definition of such a diverse and dynamic field, the emerging initiatives that adopt and adapt a community psychology approach share a certain way of understanding and responding to mental distress. In particular, community psychology approaches maintain that a person's health and happiness, as well as their difficulties and distress, can only fully be understood through an appreciation of the social context in which that person is situated. This context not only includes an individual's family, peer groups and educational or work settings, as well as their neighbourhood and geographical location, but it also extends to the 'communities of identity' with which a person associates (based on, for example, gender, class and ethnicity) and the national and even global environment within which their life is lived (Rappaport 1977; Moritsugu *et al.* 2016). In recognising how a range of social determinants can contribute to mental distress, community psychology therefore emphasises the need for interventions beyond the individual and their immediate interpersonal relationships. Rather than seeking to address a person's experience of mental distress by focusing upon the supposedly individual psychological deficits that have led to its development, community psychology shifts the focus onto the deficits within an individual's environment. In doing so, it proposes that the alleviation of a person's distress requires interventions and productive trans-formations of the social, economic and environmental conditions that can contribute to such distress.

CONCEPT SUMMARY: COMMUNITY PSYCHOLOGY INTERVENTIONS

As a result of their diverse objectives and the different contexts in which they are implemented, community psychology interventions can take various forms. While they can involve large-scale community projects, they often take the form of small-scale and predominately group-based community activities (Holmes 2015). Such activities often occur in non-mental health care settings in order to move away from the individualistic approaches that characterise mental health services, and are run by those who have experience of mental distress and by practitioners who are sympathetic to a community psychology approach. Moreover, rather than bringing people together on the basis of a shared psychiatric diagnosis, psychological dysfunction or 'mental disorder', these community psychology activities are commonly organised around people's interests, concerns and experiences of the mental health system.

While some community psychology interventions are focused upon helping people gain respite from environments that are experienced as stressful, others are more explicitly political and seek to explore the theoretical and therapeutic limitations of various aspects of contemporary mental health care. This can include education, discussion and debate about the legitimacy of psychiatric diagnoses, the effectiveness of psychiatric drugs and the social factors that can contribute to mental distress. While they can be an end in themselves, these community psychology interventions commonly encourage people to move from critique to social action. In particular, by fostering productive relationships and alliances with others who have similar concerns, these activities seek to challenge and change the individualistic orientation of mental health care in favour of social and material approaches to mental distress.

Although community psychology approaches are associated with a diverse range of interventions at a variety of levels, one of the most critical activities is the attempt to foster what has variously been referred to as 'knowing', 'outsight' or 'conscientisation' (Freire 1970; Orford 2008; Nelson & Prilleltensky 2010). To understand this activity and recognise its significance for the manner in which community psychology approaches understand and respond to mental distress, it is productive to contrast outsight with the attempt to facilitate insight that is often associated with the individualistic orientation of various psychological therapies (Castonguay & Hill 2007). By maintaining theoretical assumptions that locate the emergence and maintenance of mental distress within the individual, it has been suggested that one of the principal aims of many psychotherapeutic approaches is to invite or encourage those who experience mental distress to understand that experience in individualistic terms. That is, a principal aim of those psychological therapies that locate mental distress within the individual is to foster an intellectual or emotional self-awareness that such distress is primarily a consequence of, and perpetuated by, that individual's own psychological processes. Indeed, the ability to achieve such supposed insight and self-understanding into mental distress is often understood as a precondition for being able to make the psychological adjustments that are necessary to begin to resolve that distress (Al-Shawi 2011; Smail 2015).

In contrast with the attempt to facilitate insight, however, community psychology approaches seek to foster outsight where this involves the development of an awareness of how mental distress can be a consequence of a variety of social determinants. That is, while those psychological approaches that have an individualistic orientation seek to foster an awareness of how mental distress is primarily located within the individual, community psychology approaches attempt to facilitate an awareness of how the origins and maintenance of that distress can be located outside or beyond the individual. Therefore, while the individualistic focus of various psychological therapies is said to obscure or mystify how social factors can contribute to mental distress, it has been suggested that community psychology approaches are concerned with demystifying these factors (Smail 2014). By using productive spatial metaphors such as the power horizon, community psychology approaches not only attempt to disclose how mental distress can be a consequence of those proximal social determinants that often exist within the horizon of everyday perception and comprehension – such as low-paid employment, insecure living conditions and poor quality neighbourhoods. Rather, such approaches also seek to reveal how mental distress can be a consequence of, and maintained by, those often neglected distal social determinants which often exist beyond the horizon of everyday perception and comprehension – such as policy decisions on health and welfare expenditure, the availability of affordable housing and levels of wealth inequality throughout society.

ACTIVITY 5.5   CRITICAL THINKING

For this activity reflect upon the attempt to foster outsight as an alternative to the traditional psychotherapeutic practice of facilitating insight. As you do so, critically consider what might be the potential benefits of enabling people to understand how a variety of social and material factors may have contributed to their experience of mental distress.

An outline answer is provided at the end of the chapter.

CONCEPT SUMMARY: MORALISM

By emphasising the way in which a person's difficulties and distress can only fully be understood through an appreciation of the social context in which that individual is situated, community psychology approaches seek to draw attention to, and guard against, what is referred to as moralism in psychotherapy. In particular, community psychology maintains that by locating the origin of distress within the individual, and thereby obscuring how social factors can contribute to such distress, the individualistic focus of various psychological therapies can be associated with a tendency to engage in **victim blaming** and holding the individual responsible for the development and continuation of that distress (Ryan 1971; Nelson & Prilleltensky 2010). Therefore, as Orford (2008) has made clear, 'It is an important part of community psychology *to bring critical attention to the way in which analyses and interventions may compound distress by blaming individual or family* victims for problems that are a consequence of the way society is arranged' (p. xii, original emphasis).

As well as being associated with a tendency to hold the individual responsible for mental distress, it has also been suggested that the individualistic focus of psychological therapies can be associated with a tendency to maintain that the individual is responsible for resolving that distress. While therapeutic change is facilitated by the actions of the therapist, the ability to successfully implement that change is said to be dependent upon the client's 'self-efficacy' or 'will-power', where this is understood as an internal quality or characteristic (Smail 2014). However, while community psychology approaches maintain that the capacity to change depends upon power, the amount of power that can be exercised by an individual in any given situation is not simply a matter of the qualities possessed by that individual. Rather, it also depends upon a range of broader social factors and material conditions, including a person's financial resources, their membership of dominant social and cultural groups and the strength of that individual's social ties and connections.

CHAPTER SUMMARY

This chapter has examined a variety of critical issues surrounding the use of psychological therapies in contemporary mental health care. While a diversity of such interventions is used to respond to mental distress, we have considered their effectiveness and whether they produce beneficial outcomes for those who receive and engage with them. In the context of the dominance of some forms of psychological intervention, this chapter has also considered whether any one specific form of therapy is more effective than any other and how the quality of the therapeutic relationship, and the variety of relational factors that comprise that relationship, can influence this effectiveness. Moreover, despite the diverse range of available psychological therapies, we have considered the manner in which many of them possess an individualistic orientation in so far they seek to facilitate change within the individual. In doing so, it has been suggested that understanding and responding to mental distress in terms of this individualistic orientation has significant social and political implications, as well as potential limitations. Finally, in contrast to the individualistic focus of various psychological therapies, this chapter has discussed how a variety of emerging initiatives, both within and beyond the mental health system, can be understood as being consistent with the field of practice that is known as community psychology. In particular, it has examined the way in which community psychology interventions can be employed to understand and respond to the manner in which a variety of social and material conditions can contribute to the emergence and maintenance of mental distress.

ACTIVITIES: BRIEF OUTLINE ANSWERS

ACTIVITY 5.2 TEAM WORKING

In considering the effect of the therapeutic relationship, the client's favourable expectations, psychotherapeutic techniques and extra-therapeutic events upon successful therapeutic change, you may have had stimulating discussions with your colleagues that were informed by your clinical experiences and additional reading. However, you may have found it a particular challenge to reach a consensus about the effect of those factors in percentage terms and even questioned the ability to quantify a phenomenon as complex as psychotherapeutic change. Indeed, in acknowledging the complexity of the therapeutic encounter, and the limitations associated with quantifying the effects of psychotherapeutic factors in percentage terms, it has been suggested that such percentages ought to be understood as 'crude estimates, not as exact numbers' (Norcross & Lambert 2011, p. 12).

Despite such limitations and challenges, one of the most well-established estimates, based on thousands of outcome studies and hundreds of meta-analyses, suggests that specific psychotherapeutic techniques account for 15 per cent of the success of psychotherapeutic change. Similarly, the client's favourable expectations that the psychological intervention will be a productive and beneficial experience accounts for approximately 15 per cent of the positive influence of psychological interventions. In contrast, the therapeutic relationship has been found to account for 30 per cent while it has been estimated that extra-therapeutic events (such as a person's spontaneous remission, self-change, social support and fortuitous events) account for 40 per cent of successful psychotherapeutic change (Norcross & Lambert 2011, pp. 12–13).

ACTIVITY 5.3 REFLECTION

The attempt to determine what a cognitive behavioural approach to Vasile's mental distress might be able to achieve, and what might be its limitations, is a particularly challenging task. However, from the information given in the case study you may have considered that this form of psychological therapy might help Vasile to identify, challenge and potentially change his thoughts about his current situation and his evaluations of himself as worthless and a failure. You may also have suggested that such a process might have a beneficial effect upon his self-esteem, his feelings of self-worth and his mental health in general, and this could contribute to the development of a 'psychological resilience' conducive to his continued search for alternative employment.

You might also have considered, however, that by maintaining an individualistic orientation that is primarily concerned with facilitating change in a person's thoughts and beliefs, cognitive behavioural therapy is largely ineffective in addressing the social factors that Vasile identifies as contributing to his mental distress. Thus, you may have suggested that such an approach cannot (and indeed is not designed to) facilitate change in the working conditions under which Vasile is currently employed, the effect of that employment upon his current financial difficulties, and the economic strategy to 'maximise efficiency' that might have led to the loss of his previous job and which may be determining the low paid, insecure character of his present employment.

ACTIVITY 5.5 CRITICAL THINKING

While the successful attempt to foster outsight is dependent upon a variety of factors (such as the form of mental distress that a person is experiencing and the character of the therapeutic alliance that is established with that person), it has been suggested that it can have a variety of benefits (Orford 2008; Smail 2015). For example, outsight can help a person make a more balanced assessment of the social factors that may have contributed to their mental distress, and thus minimise the tendency for that individual to hold themselves responsible for such distress – which is said to be a potential risk associated with attempts to facilitate insight and locate mental distress within the individual.

In addition, by enabling people to consider what social and material factors may have contributed to their mental distress, outsight can also enable a person to determine what resources they currently possess, what resources they might need and what assistance they require in order to productively respond to that distress. Moreover, in so far as the facilitation of outsight is often conducted with others, it can create a sense of solidarity with those who experience similar social and material conditions, and this can form the basis for collaborative and communal action to potentially challenge, influence and even change those conditions in ways that are more conducive to people's psychological well-being.

FURTHER READING

- **Orford J** (2008) *Community Psychology: Challenges, Controversies, and Emerging Consensus*. Chichester: John Wiley & Sons.

This is an accessible and comprehensive account of community psychology with particular emphasis given to how such approaches understand and respond to the disempowerment created by social injustice and inequality.

- **Proctor G** (2017) *The Dynamics of Power in Counselling and Psychotherapy: Ethics, Politics and Practice,* 2nd edition. Monmouth: PCCS Books.

By drawing upon theories of power from a variety of academic disciplines, this book provides a thought-provoking examination of the dynamics of power within the psychotherapeutic relationship.

- **Smail D** (2014) *Power, Interest and Psychology: Elements of a Social Materialist Understanding of Distress.* Ross-on-Wye: PCCS Books.

A concise and challenging work from one of the leading critics of psychotherapy's individualistic approach to mental distress, which argues for an alternative social and material understanding of that distress.

- **Tweedy R** (2017) (ed) *The Political Self: Understanding the Social Context for Mental Illness.* London: Karnac Books.

With contributions from a range of scholars, this book provides a stimulating exploration of the relationship between mental distress and the social, political and economic context in which such distress occurs.

- **Wampold BE & Imel ZE** (2015) *The Great Psychotherapy Debate: The Evidence for What Makes Psychotherapy Work,* 2nd edition. Hove: Routledge.

An examination of the evidence for the effectiveness of psychotherapy that considers whether it is a result of specific techniques associated with certain psychotherapeutic approaches or non-specific, relational factors that are common to all.

USEFUL WEBSITES

- www.goodtherapy.org

Here you will find the website for the Good Therapy Network which works to ensure people have a positive experience with psychological therapies, and, among other things, provides a comprehensive inventory of the different types of therapy.

- www.scra27.org

This is the website for the Society for Community Research and Action, which provides information, and engages in various educational and practical activities, to promote the field of community psychology.

6

SERVICE USER/SURVIVOR INVOLVEMENT

CHAPTER AIMS

By the end of this chapter you will be able to:

- appraise service user/survivor experiences of mental health services;
- evaluate the diverse objectives of the service user/survivor movement;
- debate the involvement of service users/survivors in mental health services.

INTRODUCTION

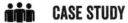 **CASE STUDY**

Aidan and his mental health colleagues are currently at an event about service user/survivor involvement in mental health services that has been organised by those who have used or who continue to use those services. During the event, Aidan has taken the opportunity to listen to service users/survivors discuss a variety of topics including their varied experiences of the mental health system and the challenges that they have encountered in seeking to effect substantial change of that system. Reflecting upon his experience of the event with his colleagues, Aidan has suggested that it has provided him with a thought-provoking perspective on the experiences of those who use mental health services and their involvement in the development, delivery and evaluation of those services. In particular, he maintains that it has reinforced his belief that it is no longer tenable for the mental health system to minimise the experiences of service users/survivors or to marginalise their attempts to question, challenge and seek to change that system.

The individual and collective involvement of people who use mental health services in the development, delivery and evaluation of those services has become one of the most significant features of contemporary mental health care. A commitment to involve service users/survivors is often reflected in the principles and policies that guide mental health practice and people who have used or who continue to use mental health services are increasingly engaged in a wide range of service activities. For example, service users/survivors are often consulted about their experiences by those who provide mental health services, and such consultancy work not only involves the monitoring and evaluation of existing services but may also contribute to the development of new services. Moreover, increasingly acknowledged as being 'experts by experience', those who use mental health services also participate in the recruitment and training of mental health professionals and, among others things, are involved in promoting alternative ways of understanding and responding to mental distress. In addition, service users/survivors are engaged in conducting research pertinent to all aspects of contemporary mental health care, and this not only involves contributing to research that is conducted by mental health professionals, but, increasingly, there is a focus on the development of user/survivor-led research. Indeed, as Aidan indicates in the above case study, it is now becoming untenable for any significant discussions about the development, delivery and evaluation of mental health services to occur without ensuring the involvement of service users/survivors in those discussions (Campbell 2013).

Despite becoming an established feature of contemporary mental health care, a variety of critical issues surround the involvement of service users/survivors in the provision of mental health services. In seeking to introduce you to these issues this chapter will begin by considering the experiences of people who have used mental health services and the significance of the personal stories or narratives that they have produced as a result. In particular, it will examine the range of concerns that service users/survivors have about the mental health system and which have motivated their demands for substantial reform of that system. We shall then discuss how the personal experiences and narratives of those who have used mental health services have been influential in the formation of service user/survivor groups that can be understood as comprising a new type of social movement. In doing so, the varied objectives and activities of this movement will be considered, along with its concern to question, challenge and seek to change any approach to mental distress which frames that experience in terms of some form of individual weakness, deficiency or disorder. Finally, while the requirement to involve service users/survivors in all aspects of mental health care is regarded as a significant achievement, this chapter will examine the ongoing critical issues surrounding the character of this involvement. In particular, it will consider the extent to which it can be understood as meaningful, rather than simply being tokenistic, as well as the variety of barriers that may obstruct the inclusive, collaborative and transformative involvement of people in mental health services.

THE EXPERIENCES OF SERVICE USERS/SURVIVORS

👥 CASE STUDY

Philippa is a mental health professional who has just attended a teaching session that was facilitated by Winston who described himself as 'a survivor of the psychiatric system'. During the course of the session, Winston discussed a variety of critical issues surrounding the use of psychiatric diagnosis, psychiatric drugs and interventions such as seclusion and restraint. Philippa was particularly struck by what he referred to as the 'disempowering consequences' of receiving a psychiatric diagnosis and his account of the 'dehumanising and coercive practices' to which he has been subjected. In particular, Philippa is beginning to consider that she has until now given minimal consideration to the first-hand experience of being in the mental health system. While she has acquired a body of professional knowledge about the various theoretical and therapeutic approaches that are employed in mental health care, she has minimal knowledge of the experiences of those who use mental health services and the concerns that they may have about those services.

Over the past thirty years, the personal experiences and narratives of those who have used mental health services have provided powerful, challenging and sometimes even disturbing accounts of the mental health system (Chamberlin 1978; Read & Reynolds 1996; Russo & Sweeney 2016). Of course, mental health systems are large, complex and multifaceted entities, and one individual's experience of that system can differ markedly from the experience of another individual. For example, the experience of a person who has been given a diagnosis of schizophrenia and who has had repeated involuntarily admissions to a mental health hospital will be significantly different from someone who has experienced a period of anxiety and who has been taking prescribed medication and receiving psychotherapy in a community-based mental health setting. Despite this variance, however, what unifies many of the personal experiences and narratives of those who have used mental health services is an overriding sense that, in the main, they have not been well served by the mental health system. Indeed, while the service user/survivor movement is characterised by a diversity of aims, values and beliefs, one of its central unifying themes and motivating factors has been the negative experiences of those who have used or who continue to use mental health services. As Campbell (2012) has noted, 'it remains true that shared memories of personal mistreatment at the hands of mental health workers are powerful cohesive elements in the movement. Legends of oppression met and overcome are important parts of the service user/survivor culture' (p. 198).

While the negative experiences of those who use mental health services vary considerably, they have contributed to an image of a mental health system that is inconsistent or fragmented at best and, at worst, is ineffective, intimidating and detrimental to a person's well-being. For example, there can be long delays in accessing appropriate mental health services and when those services are accessed people can experience a pressure to resolve or recover from their distress and disengage from services before they feel ready to do so (Beresford 2010). In addition, those who use mental health services report feeling unsafe, threatened and even traumatised by witnessing or being subject to a range of distressing events that can occur in mental health settings such as verbal and physical aggression and the use of coercive measures such as seclusion, restraint and forced medication (Sweeney *et al.* 2016). Moreover, even when such explicit displays of power and control do not occur, the personal narratives of service users/survivors recount how mental health practitioners have used demeaning language, displayed discriminatory attitudes and engaged in subtle forms of persuasion and coercion to ensure compliance with treatment (Gonzales *et al.* 2015; Sweeney *et al.* 2015). As a consequence, it has been suggested that the mental health system can often feel like an additional obstacle that those experiencing mental distress have to endure, navigate and survive, rather than a provider of safe and effective care that is responsive to the interests, concerns and needs of those who use mental health services (Beresford 2010).

───── CONCEPT SUMMARY: EXPERIENTIAL KNOWLEDGE ─────

The knowledge that informs the provision of mental health care originates from a variety of sources and is produced by using a diversity of means. In part influenced by the requirement to provide evidence-based practice in mental health care, knowledge that is produced by certain means (such as the use of **quantitative research methodologies** and randomised controlled trials in particular) has commonly been valued more highly than knowledge produced by other means (Guyatt *et al.* 2015). In prioritising certain forms of knowledge production, particular emphasis has been placed upon the need to limit the influence of personal experience on all aspects of the research process and thereby produce knowledge that is supposedly impersonal, unbiased and universal. Measured against such standards, the personal experiences and narratives of those who use mental health services have often been devalued and even dismissed as being partial, biased and anecdotal (Faulkner 2017).

In challenging such assessments, the service user/survivor movement prioritises the personal experiences of those who use mental health services and emphasises the value of the insights, evidence and knowledge which these experiences can provide. Indeed, the attempt to adopt a position of neutrality in the research process is not only considered to be untenable but is also said to produce knowledge that can distort attempts to productively understand and respond to the 'lived experience' of mental distress (Wallcraft 2015; Beresford 2016). Moreover, while the experiential knowledge of service users/survivors is invariably grounded in personal experience, it has been suggested that it need not necessarily be limited to that experience (Sweeney 2016). Rather, by robustly adopting certain **qualitative research methodologies** such as **autoethnography**, attention can be given to the way in which a person's experience intersects with the experiences of others and provides wider cultural, social and political insights into mental distress.

ACTIVITY 6.1 RESEARCH

The various forms of inquiry, investigation and research into all aspects of mental distress, primarily conducted by service users/survivors, have developed considerably over the last twenty years (Rose 2001; Sweeney *et al.* 2009; Staddon 2015).

Most recently, there has been an interest in the way in which this work has become manifest within, and made productive connections with, the emerging field of inquiry known as Mad Studies (Sweeney 2016; Faulkner 2017).

For this activity conduct your own investigations into Mad Studies and attempt to provide a concise definition of this emerging and dynamic field, as well as an overview of its characteristic features and primary concerns.

An outline answer is provided at the end of the chapter.

Although service user/survivor narratives have highlighted a variety of ways in which the mental health system has not adequately met the needs of those who experience mental distress, a fundamental concern has been with the manner in which that distress is framed or understood. That is, one of the most consistent themes to emerge from those narratives is that the biological or biomedical model continues to dominate the way in which mental health professionals understand and respond to the experience of mental distress (Campbell 2012; Beresford *et al.* 2016). In doing so, those who use mental health services commonly report that their experiences have been framed in medical terms and have been understood as the manifestation of some form of individual and predominately biological dysfunction. As a consequence, many service users/survivors maintain that at some point during their engagement with the mental health system they have accepted and internalised this biological approach (Cohen & Hughes 2011; Beresford *et al.* 2016). Moreover, some people report that doing so, at least initially, was a source of comfort, relief and reassurance in so far as it provided a seemingly accessible and convincing explanation for the confusing and sometimes disturbing experiences that were associated with their mental distress. However, many service users/survivors maintain that the way in which their experiences have been understood as some form of individual and predominately biological dysfunction, and the manner in which they have experienced a pressure from mental health professionals to accept such an understanding, has been largely unhelpful, ineffective and even damaging (Beresford *et al.* 2016).

The personal narratives of service users/survivors highlight a variety of ways in which the biological approach to mental distress can have counterproductive consequences. For example, understood as a manifestation of some form of underlying biological dysfunction, the biomedical model is said to foster a reliance on psychiatric drugs as the primary response to mental distress. As discussed in Chapter 4, by uncritically accepting the short-term and long-term effectiveness of psychiatric drugs to target and correct such supposed dysfunctions, there can be a focus upon ensuring compliance with drug regimes and a limited consideration of the adverse effects of those drugs and the need for service user/survivor involvement in decisions about their use (Deegan & Drake 2006; Read 2009). Moreover, by understanding mental distress as some form of individual dysfunction, the opinions of those who use mental health services are often subordinated to the technical knowledge and judgements of practitioners. In particular, the biological approach can contribute to the marginalisation of how people make sense of their mental distress and the expertise they may have acquired as a result of seeking to understand and respond to that distress (Coles 2015). In addition, a consistent theme that emerges from the personal narratives of service users/survivors is that the biological approach to mental distress is experienced as stigmatising, discriminatory and exclusionary. In particular, by being associated with a variety of stereotypical assumptions and negative societal perceptions, those who use mental health services maintain that the biomedical model has contributed to the way in which they have been identified by others as being different, deficient and even potentially dangerous (Beresford *et al.* 2016).

ACTIVITY 6.2   RESEARCH

For this activity go to the Mad in America website and access the 'personal stories' archive (www.madinamerica.com/category/personal-stories/) where you will find narratives of people's experience of mental distress and their treatment by the mental health system.

As you explore those narratives reflect upon the range of concerns that people have about established ways of understanding and responding to mental distress and consider how their personal stories provide perspectives and insights that may not otherwise have been available to you.

As this activity is based upon your own research, there is no outline answer at the end of the chapter.

While the narratives of service users/survivors highlight how contact with the mental health system can lead to being labelled as different from other members of society, they also stress that the diversity of those who use mental health services has not been adequately recognised. Indeed, an enduring criticism of the mental health system is that it has failed to acknowledge, respect and productively respond to how people's experience of that system, and the experience of mental distress itself, can be influenced by a variety of intersecting variables such as a person's gender, race, ethnicity, age, sexual orientation, nationality, spirituality and socio-economic status. While the reasons given for this are complex and contested, service user/survivor narratives have highlighted that the traditional dominance of a biological approach to mental distress has been a significant contributory factor (Beresford *et al.* 2016). By seeking to understand and respond to the mental distress experienced by diverse groups of people as some form of biological dysfunction, the significance of that diversity has been subordinated to the common pathological processes that supposedly underlie the emergence and maintenance of such distress. As a consequence, mental health services are said to have failed to understand mental distress in the context of such diversity, and the way in which different groups of people can have significantly different experiences of the mental health system. In addition, the narratives of service users/ survivors have drawn attention to how the mental health system can reflect and reinforce the broader social inequalities and forms of discrimination that can be directed against those diverse groups.

The experience of the mental health system by people from black and minority ethnic communities, for example, is one of the most enduring critical issues in mental health care. While a variety of differences exist within and between these communities, the research indicates that, when taken as a collective, people from these communities experience significant inequalities in mental health care in comparison to the majority white community (Fitzpatrick *et al.* 2014). For example, people from black and minority ethnic communities are more likely to be compulsorily admitted to mental health services, to be treated in a secure setting, to be subject to coercive practices and to be prescribed psychiatric drugs rather than receive psychological therapies. Moreover, black and minority ethnic service users/survivors more commonly have their mental distress misunderstood and misdiagnosed, while those from African Caribbean communities are more likely to be perceived as violent or dangerous and to be given a diagnosis of schizophrenia. A number of explanations for these inequalities have been provided, including the effect of cultural differences, the increased social and economic disadvantage experienced by black and minority ethnic communities, and the psychological stress surrounding migration and **acculturation**. However, the personal experiences and narratives of people from these communities have contributed to claims that not only are such inequalities the result of the discriminatory attitudes, beliefs and behaviour of individual practitioners, but they should also be understood as a reflection of a more pervasive structural or **institutional racism** that is characteristic of the mental health system (Jackson 2002; Fernando 2008; King 2016).

· ACTIVITY 6.3   REFLECTION

The suggestion that the mental health system is institutionally racist is a controversial, challenging and complex claim that has been the subject of ongoing critical discussion (Fitzpatrick *et al.* 2014; Fernando 2017). Partly as a response to this claim, however,

(Continued)

there has been an increased demand for practitioners to provide culturally sensitive, competent and capable mental health care. Despite this, it has been suggested that cultural competence and capability training in mental health care, and the presence of culturally competent health care in general, has been inconsistent at best (Holland 2018).

For this activity reflect upon your knowledge of culturally competent mental health care, and your experience of its provision in the clinical setting, by considering the following questions:

- What teaching, training or information have you received about culturally competent mental health care?
- What evidence have you seen of culturally competent mental health care being provided in the clinical environment?
- To what extent do you feel able to provide culturally competent mental health care?

As this activity is based upon your own reflections, there is no outline answer at the end of the chapter.

CONCEPT SUMMARY: INTERSECTIONALITY

Attempts to understand and productively respond to discrimination have traditionally focused upon its singular forms, such as racism, sexism, ageism, classism, ableism, homophobia, transphobia and xenophobia. As a consequence, it has been suggested that the experiences of those who confront multiple forms of discrimination have often been marginalised or overlooked. In seeking to challenge this omission, the notion of intersectionality – introduced by the American civil rights advocate and academic Kimberlé Crenshaw (1989) – emphasises the manner in which certain individuals and groups of people can be subject to overlapping or intersecting forms of discrimination. In doing so, it maintains that these intersecting forms of discrimination, such as the racism and sexism that can be experienced by black women, constitute an experience that cannot adequately be accounted for by examining the race or gender dimensions of that experience separately.

While initially introduced to understand and challenge the failure of anti-discrimination law to recognise the combination of racism and sexism faced by black women, intersectionality has been applied to varying contexts including mental health care (Hallett 2015; Mizock & Russinova 2015). It thus enables an exploration of how service users/survivors can experience multiple forms of discrimination. In particular, rather than seeking to understand the discrimination faced by people solely on the basis of their mental distress, intersectionality highlights the importance of recognising how such discrimination can overlap and coexist with, for example, racism, sexism or homophobia. Intersectionality therefore shifts attention to those combined forms of discrimination (such as may be experienced by service users/survivors from lesbian, gay, bisexual and transgender communities) that have often been neglected by analyses of discrimination that only focus upon its singular forms.

THE SERVICE USER/SURVIVOR MOVEMENT

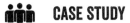 **CASE STUDY**

As part of her ongoing professional development, Isabella is conducting her own investigations into the service user/survivor movement and attempting to determine its characteristic features and primary objectives. However, she has discovered that the movement is comprised of a diversity of groups and organisations that have varying objectives and which engage in a wide range of activities to pursue those objectives. In particular, she has found out that the service user/survivor movement is not only concerned with enabling the voices of those who use mental health services to be heard in order to effect changes within those services. Rather, she has discovered that it is, for example, variously concerned with challenging the stigma, discrimination and exclusion that those who experience mental distress can encounter; with reclaiming the experience of mental distress and seeking to redefine it as a potentially meaningful experience; and with engaging in various forms of activism in order to facilitate the development of environments, communities and even whole societies that are more conducive to people's mental well-being.

The personal experiences and narratives of those who use mental health services have been powerful motivating factors in the formation of service user/survivor groups that seek to transform the provision of mental health care. However, although the emergence of these groups has been understood as a new type of social movement, it is important to recognise that a characteristic feature of this movement is its diversity. As Isabella is discovering in the above case study, a variety of service user/survivor organisations exist at the local, national and international levels and they are notable both for the range of activities in which they participate and the diverse assumptions, values and beliefs that inform those activities (Beresford 2010). While some organisations are focused upon providing direct support for those experiencing mental distress, others are more concerned with addressing the broader challenges that people who use mental health services can confront, such as stigma, discrimination and exclusion. Moreover, some groups are organised around particular experiences associated with mental distress, such as hearing voices or unusual beliefs, while others prioritise the needs of those from particular communities, such as black and minority ethnic mental health service users/survivors. In addition, service user/survivor groups have different assessments of the worth of existing mental health services and different objectives in relation to those services. For example, while some groups are working to reform the mental health system, there are others, sceptical of the possibility of meaningful involvement in that system, who are focused upon the development of separate service-user/survivor-led mental health care.

Therefore, in so far as the collective action of those who use mental health services can be understood as a new type of social movement, it is not necessarily a movement that coheres around an agreed set of aims, objectives or activities. While all service users/survivors are united in having an experience of the mental health system, they may differ in terms of their understanding of and responses to that system. Despite these differences, however, it is possible to identify a number of common positions, beliefs and activities that are shared across the diverse range of service user/survivor groups (Wallcraft *et al.* 2003). For example, they are invariably concerned with challenging the stigma, discrimination and exclusion that can be associated with mental distress, as well as being committed to increasing the opportunities for greater social inclusion for those who experience such distress. In addition, they are characteristically critical of the dominance of the biomedical model of mental distress and the associated reliance on physiological interventions such as psychiatric medication and electroconvulsive therapy. Moreover, service user/survivor groups commonly insist on the need for the experiences and expertise of those who use mental health services to be acknowledged and stress the value of service-user/survivor-led interventions such as peer support, mentoring and befriending. Finally, those groups are almost universally opposed to the extension of compulsory powers to detain people who experience mental distress, as well as being concerned to ensure the reduction, and in many cases elimination, of coercive practices such as seclusion, restraint and forced medication.

ACTIVITY 6.4   TEAM WORKING

Although the use of coercive practices has been an enduring feature of mental health care, it has been suggested that how such practices are experienced by those who use mental health services, and the effect that they have on treatment outcomes, has been given minimal consideration (Luciano *et al.* 2014; McLaughlin *et al.* 2016).

For this activity reflect with your colleagues upon the possible effects of coercive measures such as seclusion, restraint and forced medication. In particular, attempt to provide an account of the ways in which those measures might be experienced by service users/survivors and their potential effects on treatment outcomes.

An outline answer is provided at the end of the chapter.

While the variety of groups and organisations that comprise the service user/survivor movement share a number of common positions, one of the most fundamental concerns has been to 'reclaim' and redefine the experience of mental distress (Campbell 2013; Russo 2016). Against the frameworks and models that have been promoted by mental health professionals and that have dominated how mental distress has been understood, the service user/survivor movement has characteristically asserted the right of those who use mental health services to understand their experiences in their own terms. Of all the professionally devised and endorsed approaches to mental distress that service user/survivor groups have challenged, the greatest opposition has been directed against the biomedical model and the associated practice of psychiatric diagnosis. In doing so, those groups have not only focused attention on and campaigned against the potentially stigmatising consequences of receiving a psychiatric diagnosis, but have also consistently challenged the notion that such diagnoses identify biologically based medical 'illnesses'. Furthermore, rather than being exclusively concerned with the biomedical model, the service user/survivor movement has resisted any approach to mental distress which understands that experience as the manifestation of some form of individual dysfunction or deficit, irrespective of whether that supposed deficit is understood in biological or psychological terms. In doing so, the concern to reclaim and redefine the experience of mental distress has been closely associated with a vigorous rejection of any framework that either directly or indirectly leads people to believe that their distress is the result of some form of individual weakness, deficiency or disorder that differentiates them from others.

Against what it regards as the predominately pathologising professional frameworks that have dominated mental health care, the service user/survivor movement has been influential in developing a range of alternative approaches – such as those associated with the hearing voices movement and with trauma-informed approaches to mental distress (Corstens *et al.* 2014; Sweeney *et al.* 2016). As highlighted in Chapter 2, rather than being understood as the largely meaningless manifestation of some form of individual dysfunction, these approaches maintain that mental distress can be a potentially meaningful experience. In particular, the underlying assumption of these alternative approaches is that the thoughts, feelings and behaviour which can be associated with mental distress, no matter how complex, unusual or disturbing they are, can on some level be understood as making sense once they are situated in the unique context of a person's life history and current circumstances. However, while the service user/survivor movement has characteristically asserted the value of these alternative approaches over those that have dominated mental health care, it has not sought universal acceptance for one single approach to mental distress. Rather, there has been a recognition that reclaiming the experience of mental distress should mean that each service user/survivor is at liberty to define their individual experience in a way that they find personally productive. While some people may choose to reject the professional frameworks that have dominated how mental distress has been understood, others may not, and there is an acknowledgement within the service user/survivor movement that such a decision should be respected (Russo 2016).

PRACTICE ISSUE: SELF-INJURY

The narratives of those who engage in acts of self-harm or self-injury, such as cutting, burning or abrading, have been influential in challenging established ways of understanding and responding to those acts (Pembroke 1995; Cresswell 2005). For example, self-injury has often been discussed in the context of and even conflated with suicide, whereas service

(Continued)

user/survivor narratives have maintained a clear distinction between the two. In particular, people are said to engage in suicidal behaviours in order to end their lives, often because they feel as though they are no longer able to cope with and continue those lives. In contrast, service user/survivor narratives highlight that self-injury serves a variety of functions related to coping with and preserving life in the presence of various adversities such as physical, sexual and emotional abuse, feelings of guilt and self-hatred and issues surrounding sexual orientation (Shaw 2016).

Rather than being understood as a dysfunctional and meaningless act, service user/survivor narratives have therefore presented self-injury as an embodied response to mental distress that can be understood as meaningful once it is situated in the biographical context of a person's life and current circumstances (Inckle 2017). In doing so, those narratives stress the importance of a collaborative examination of the function of self-injury and the mental distress that such acts are being employed to address, as well as an exploration of less harmful ways of responding to that distress. In this context, self-injury is not understood as the manifestation of some form of individual weakness, deficiency or disorder but as belonging to a continuum of strategies, some more constructive and socially acceptable than others, that people use to cope with and survive difficult feelings, emotions and circumstances (Sutton 2007).

In being concerned with reclaiming and redefining the experience of mental distress, the service user/survivor movement has not only been influential in developing approaches that seek to facilitate an exploration of the personal meaning of that distress, it has also supported and contributed to the development of social models and approaches to mental distress. As we discussed in Chapter 2, these approaches share the assumption that, rather than being understood as the manifestation of some form of individual dysfunction, the experiences of service users/survivors ought to be situated in a wider social, economic and political context. In particular, they highlight how a variety of factors that are located outside or beyond the individual can profoundly influence the social and material conditions of people's lives and, in doing so, contribute to the emergence and maintenance of mental distress throughout the course of those lives (Compton & Shim 2015). In promoting social approaches to mental distress, however, the service user/survivor movement has not only been concerned with the manner in which those proximal social determinants such as insecure employment, poor housing and low-quality neighbourhoods can contribute to mental distress; rather, it has also focused attention on the relationship between mental distress and a range of distal social determinants such as local and national decisions on health and welfare expenditure, the occurrence of economic recessions and levels of wealth inequality throughout society, and even the suggested 'maddening' character of the communities, societies and world in which people live (Beresford 2010; Beresford *et al.* 2016).

By situating the experiences associated with mental distress in their wider social, economic and political contexts, the service user/survivor movement has therefore not confined its concerns to the perceived failings of the mental health system. Rather, it has consistently highlighted the ways in which those who use mental health services can confront a variety of challenges beyond those services, including various forms of social exclusion, discrimination and oppression (Thornicroft 2006; Campbell 2013). In doing so, the service user/survivor movement has not been content simply to analyse and draw attention to those challenges, but has characteristically participated in various forms of activism in an attempt to address them. In particular, many of the groups and organisations that comprise the service user/survivor movement have been actively involved in seeking to ensure that those who experience mental distress have the same access to the range of life opportunities that are afforded to other members of society. Given the challenges involved in attempting to secure such objectives, the service user/survivor movement has increasingly sought to forge productive alliances with other marginalised groups and progressive social movements that have confronted and attempted to address various forms of exclusion, discrimination and oppression (LeFrançois *et al.* 2013). In doing so, there has been a concern to learn from the work of these groups and social movements in order to develop social approaches to mental distress that can facilitate the creation of environments, communities and whole societies that are more conducive to the well-being of those who use mental health services.

CONCEPT SUMMARY: THE SOCIAL MODEL OF DISABILITY

While originally developed by the **disabled people's movement**, there has been increased interest in how the social model of disability might enable an alternative and potentially productive social approach to mental distress. In doing so, this model draws a distinction between an impairment (or a perceived impairment) and a disability. While the former refers to an aspect of a person's physical, sensory or intellectual capabilities, the latter designates the negative societal responses to that person's particular impairment (Oliver 2013; Beresford *et al.* 2016). Rather than being an attribute of the individual, disability is therefore understood in terms of the discriminatory, oppressive and exclusionary responses that people with an impairment can confront. As such, the social model of disability seeks to address those disabling social responses in order to provide people who have an impairment with access to the range of opportunities that are afforded to other members of society.

It has therefore been suggested that the social model of disability provides a productive framework in which to situate the experiences of those who use mental health services (Beresford 2016). In contrast to those approaches that understand and respond to mental distress as some form of individual dysfunction, the social model of disability can be used to consider, challenge and seek to change the discriminatory and disabling social responses that those who use mental health services can experience from others. However, while some service users/survivors have acknowledged the potential significance of this model in the context of mental distress, others have expressed reservations. In particular, there has been a reluctance to understand any aspect of the experience of mental distress by using terms such as disability and impairment, and a concern that doing so would reinforce perceptions of mental distress as some form of personal weakness, deficiency or dysfunction (Campbell 2012; Beresford *et al.* 2016).

THE MEANINGFUL INVOLVEMENT OF SERVICE USERS/SURVIVORS

CASE STUDY

Stuart and Rashida are reflecting upon their recent experiences of attending mental health service development meetings in their capacity as users of those services. Despite concerns about the terminology used in the meetings, Stuart suggests that he found his involvement a largely positive experience. In particular, he felt that he was able to raise a variety of issues pertinent to service users/survivors over the course of the meetings and that his contribution appeared to be valued by the other participants. In contrast, Rashida suggests that her experience was less positive. Although the meetings were supposedly a forum to discuss the development of services, she received the impression that the major decisions had already been taken and she was there simply to approve them. Moreover, despite attempting to raise a number of issues, Rashida says she was variously told that the meetings 'were not the appropriate forum' to do so, that those issues 'may be considered' at some other time, and, on one occasion, that she was 'not representative' of the majority of those who use mental health services.

The involvement of people who use mental health services in various aspects of the development, delivery and evaluation of those services is now an established feature of contemporary mental health care. As Campbell (2013) has suggested, 'Service users have a voice in every mental health sector ... they are now a presence in aspects of mental health services in which their presence would have been inconceivable a quarter of a century ago; this is an indication of the change in climate that has occurred' (p. 140). As illustrated in the above case study, however, there are ongoing critical concerns about the character of this involvement and the degree to which it can be understood as meaningful rather than simply being **tokenistic**. For example, questions exist about whether the varying objectives of the service user/survivor movement have been achieved or are likely to be achieved in the context of existing mental health services. In addition, there have been related concerns about the influence and power that people possess, or are permitted to possess, in order to effect substantial change within the mental health system. Moreover, while service user/survivor groups are commonly involved in discussions about the provision of mental health care, there are ongoing questions about the extent to which this has empowered the individuals who use those services and the degree to which they participate in the planning and delivery of their own care and treatment (Wallcraft *et al.* 2003; Bee *et al.* 2015; Faulkner *et al.* 2015).

While it is commonly acknowledged that the requirement to involve service users/survivors in all aspects of mental health care has been a significant achievement, it has also been suggested that a variety of barriers exist within the mental health system which can obstruct greater degrees of meaningful involvement. Indeed, it has been proposed that these barriers can not only impede the ongoing involvement of people in the provision of mental health services, but they can also actively discourage those service users/survivors who might otherwise have become involved (Beresford 2013). For example, those who have experience of participating in various forms of service user/survivor involvement commonly assert that the opinions, experiences and knowledge of mental health professionals are often given greater credibility than the opinions, experiences and knowledge of those who use mental health services. Moreover, it has been suggested that there is a resistance to critical concerns about the dominance of the biomedical model and the associated reliance on psychiatric drugs, as well as a suspicion of those alternative approaches to mental distress that have been developed and are promoted by the service user/ survivor movement. In addition, an over-reliance on jargon and technical language, a lack of appropriate and readily available information, inflexible and bureaucratic organisational systems, as well as insufficient resources and obstacles surrounding the financial costs of participation, have all been identified as restricting the mean-ingful involvement of people who use mental health services in the development, delivery and evaluation of those services (Hitchen *et al.* 2011; Campbell 2013).

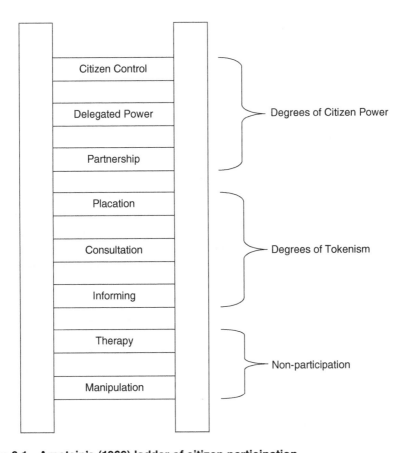

Figure 6.1   Arnstein's (1969) ladder of citizen participation

------ **PRACTICE ISSUE: ARNSTEIN'S LADDER OF PARTICIPATION** ------

In differentiating the various forms that user/survivor involvement in mental health services can take, and attempting to determine the degree to which that involvement can be understood as meaningful, it can be productive to think in terms of a 'ladder of participation'. While initially developed to distinguish levels of citizen participation in various areas, one of the most influential ladders for thinking about user/survivor involvement in health care is that developed by Sherry Arnstein (1969) (Figure 6.1).

In presenting eight rungs or levels of citizen participation, Arnstein identifies *manipulation* and *therapy* as the least participatory and influential forms of involvement. While providing opportunities that give the appearance of participation (such as being invited to attend various meetings about service provision), at these levels of involvement service users/survivors are informed about the way in which services are currently provided and then expected, manipulated or coerced into simply endorsing those services.

The next levels of participation are referred to as *informing*, *consultation* and *placation* and variously involve providing service users/survivors with information about their rights, seeking their opinions and ideas and appointing user/survivor representatives to influential committees. However, while these forms of involvement give people a voice in the provision of services, Arnstein maintains that they remain largely tokenistic in so far as there is no genuine commitment to heed that voice and change services as a result.

The higher forms of involvement that Arnstein identifies are referred to as *partnership*, *delegated power* and *citizen control* in which users/survivors have increasing degrees of meaningful influence over the provision of services. These levels of participation involve becoming equal partners in decision-making processes, being given the power to effect substantial reform of particular services and, at the topmost level, having full managerial control over certain services and the conditions under which they can be changed.

To facilitate greater degrees of meaningful user/survivor involvement in mental health services, it has been suggested that more needs to be done to remove the barriers that can obstruct such involvement. In doing so, the concern should not simply be to enable involvement in the existing provision of services, which, it is argued, places people in a subordinate position in relation to those services; rather, the focus ought to be on co-production, in which professionals and service users/survivors become equal partners in the development and delivery of those services (Slay & Stephens 2013; Clark 2015). While the means used to facilitate such participation will be specific to the particular context in which it is sought, a variety of standards, strategies and initiatives have been proposed to promote more inclusive, collaborative and transformative user/survivor involvement (Beresford 2013; Faulkner *et al.* 2015; Carr & Patel 2016). For example, it has been suggested that mental health services need to become more proactive in providing people with information about how to become involved as well as ensuring that service users/survivors from a diversity of backgrounds have access to such involvement. Moreover, people who use mental health services need to be provided with the opportunity to be present at all stages and levels of the decision-making process, and to be active in the development of care provision rather than just its delivery. In addition, it has been suggested that there needs to be a greater emphasis on providing people with practical, emotional and financial support in order to actively encourage user/survivor participation in services and to increase the likelihood of that participation being sustained and becoming established.

Central to the development of meaningful service user/survivor involvement, however, is a recognition of, and a commitment to address, the imbalances in power, influence and status that exist between those who use mental health services and those who currently provide those services (Beresford 2013; Faulkner *et al.* 2015). While a variety of practical initiatives can assist in the development of more equitable relationships between those two groups, a significant shift is required in the attitudes, values and beliefs towards people who use mental health services and the experience of mental distress more generally. For example, rather than being understood as the manifestation of some form of individual biological or psychological dysfunction, a widespread receptivity to understanding mental distress as a potentially meaningful experience is needed, as well as an associated concern with the strengths and capabilities that people possess, or can develop, as a consequence of that experience. In turn, this will require a greater degree of humility with respect to the professionally developed and endorsed approaches to mental distress that have come to dominate mental health care and a willingness to engage with those alternative, non-medicalised approaches that are supported by the service user/survivor movement. Moreover, addressing the power differentials within mental health services, and thereby facilitating more meaningful user/survivor involvement, will require that the personal experience of mental distress is understood as a legitimate form of knowing that can enable insights into understanding and responding to that distress which may not be available by other means.

ACTIVITY 6.5   RESEARCH

One of the most profound obstacles to the establishment of more equitable relationships in contemporary mental health care is the manner in which service users/survivors can be subject to **epistemic injustice**.

For this activity conduct your own research into the notion of epistemic injustice and attempt to determine its meaning as well as its significance for those who use mental health services. An outline answer is provided at the end of the chapter.

Despite the variety of challenges that they can confront, many service users/survivors remain committed to questioning, challenging and seeking to effect substantial change in the mental health system. However, there is a belief among some of those who comprise the service user/survivor movement that, rather than seeking to reform existing mental health services, the concern should be with the development and delivery of user-controlled services. While the reasons for establishing such services will be specific to the individuals, groups and organisations involved, an enduring concern has been with the imbalances in power that persist within the mental health system, and, in particular, the manner in which service user/survivor involvement in that system can be co-opted (Chamberlin 1978; Penny & Prescott 2016). In the context of mental health care, **co-option** refers to the variety of ways in which the mental health system can take over or assimilate the theoretical and therapeutic innovations introduced by service users/survivors, and, in the process, remove or neutralise aspects of those innovations which challenge that system's power and authority. Therefore, in seeking to avoid the co-option of its work, and retain the independence and autonomy to pursue its own objectives, the service user/survivor movement has a history of choosing to establish its own services rather than becoming involved with existing mental health services. While they often face a variety of obstacles – such as the ongoing challenge to secure funding for their continued existence – user-controlled services can include drop-in groups and day centres, telephone and on-line forum support, safe houses and crisis houses, and various forms of mentoring services, skills training and employment projects (Beresford 2010; Lindow 2012).

User-controlled services can therefore provide a wide range of services to those who experience mental distress and they can employ a variety of theoretical, therapeutic and practical means in order to do so. Despite this variance, however, these services invariably involve people who have or who continue to experience mental distress providing support to others who experience such distress. In receiving support from their peers, those who engage with user-controlled services identify a variety of advantages over existing mental health services, such as feeling less isolated with their experience of mental distress and being able to explore it without fear of judgement, as well as being empowered to develop their own way of understanding and coping with that experience (Beresford 2010; Shaw 2015). Moreover, it has been suggested that one of the central advantages of user-controlled services is that they are more likely to facilitate the development of equitable relationships between people in comparison with existing mental health services (Chamberlin 1978). In particular, user-controlled services commonly seek to challenge the enduring distinction between 'us and them' and the associated positioning of some people as mental health 'experts' or 'professionals' with power and authority to determine how others' experience of mental distress should be understood and addressed. Indeed, when the emphasis is on people who have experience of mental distress providing support to each other, then the power imbalances that can exist between the helper and the helped can be significantly reduced and replaced with more reciprocal and mutually empowering relationships in which those who receive peer support can also be those who provide such support.

CONCEPT SUMMARY: PEER SUPPORT

The support that those who have experience of mental distress can provide to one another has taken multiple forms, either arising spontaneously between people or being conducted in a more formal, structured manner. Along with an increased interest in the potentially beneficial effects of peer support, however, there has been a concern to investigate the features that characterise effective peer relationships. Consequently, it has been suggested that important features include mutuality, equality and respect, so that people are enabled to explore how to understand and respond to their experience of mental distress in their own terms (Faulkner & Kalathil 2012). Moreover, the sharing of experiences and the mutual support that often occurs during this process can facilitate an atmosphere of empathy, trust and empowerment, in which a person's feelings of isolation, fear and pessimism about mental distress can be replaced with hope, optimism and the belief that recovery is possible (Davidson *et al.* 2012).

While the effectiveness of peer support has been disputed (Lloyd-Evans *et al.* 2014), increasing numbers of mental health services have begun to employ peer support workers. It has been suggested that in this way they can bring a range of benefits to the mental health system, such as advocating for those who experience mental distress and influencing the development and delivery of existing mental health services (Repper & Carter 2011). However, critical concerns exist about the extent to which peer support is being co-opted by those services and the manner in which the professionalisation of that role can distort its characteristic features. In particular, it has been suggested that peer support workers can experience pressure to conform to the dominant norms, values and practices of the mental health system and thereby collude in maintaining the imbalances in power, authority and status which can characterise that system (Brown & Stansy 2016; Filson & Mead 2016).

CHAPTER SUMMARY

This chapter has examined a variety of critical issues surrounding the involvement of users/survivors in the provision of mental health services. In particular, it has considered the varied experiences of those who have used mental health services and the significance of the personal stories or narratives that they have produced as a result. In doing so, it has discussed the range of concerns that service users/survivors have about the mental health system and which have motivated their demand for substantial reform of that system. Moreover, we have also highlighted how the personal experiences and narratives of those who have used mental health services have been influential in the formation of user/survivor groups, which can be understood as comprising a new type of social movement. In the process, the varied objectives and activities of this movement have been considered along with its concern to question, challenge and seek to change any approach to mental distress which frames that experience in terms of some form of individual weakness, deficiency or disorder. Finally, while the requirement to involve service users/survivors in all aspects of mental health care is regarded as a significant achievement, this chapter has concluded by examining the ongoing critical issues surrounding the character of this involvement. In particular, it has considered the extent to which it can be understood as meaningful, rather than simply being tokenistic, as well as the variety of barriers that may need to be addressed in order to facilitate more inclusive, collaborative and transformative service user/survivor involvement.

ACTIVITIES: BRIEF OUTLINE ANSWERS

ACTIVITY 6.1 RESEARCH

As a developing field of inquiry, you may have discovered that Mad Studies can be a particular challenge to define concisely. Indeed, it has been referred to as an 'in/discipline' to denote the way in which it seeks to provocatively challenge many of the assumptions and practices that have been associated with what is thought to constitute a legitimate area of study (Ingram 2016). In general terms, however, Mad Studies has been defined as a field of inquiry, a body of knowledge and a project of political engagement that is concerned with the experiences, knowledge and activism of those who have experienced or who continue to experience mental distress (Menzies *et al.* 2013). Moreover, while it is primarily focused on and conducted by those who experience mental distress, Mad Studies also makes productive alliances with other marginalised groups, as well as those academics, practitioners and activists who identify with its concerns and who work within, across and beyond traditional academic disciplines.

As a wide-ranging field of study, it has been suggested that Mad Studies is characterised by a diversity of features and objectives (Menzies *et al.* 2013). For example, it is opposed to the biomedical model of mental distress and is concerned with developing alternative approaches that situate such distress in the unique context of a person's life history and current circumstances. In addition, it seeks to confront the variety of ways in which the experiences, knowledge and expertise of those who use mental health services is commonly delegitimised, both within and beyond those services, and to address the imbalances in power, influence and status that can contribute to this condition. Moreover, it is concerned with investigating and resisting the manner in which the theoretical and therapeutic innovations introduced by service users/survivors are taken over or co-opted by the mental health system and the way in which those innovations, during this process, are appropriated and distorted by that system.

ACTIVITY 6.4 TEAM WORKING

Although it is an area that has been insufficiently researched, the available evidence indicates that coercive practices have a diverse range of effects upon those who use mental health services. For example, those who are subject to coercive practices often report feelings of humiliation, distress and violation, and there are increasing concerns about the psychological risks associated with their use and their potential to re-traumatise those who have been subject to adverse events in the past (Sibitz *et al.* 2011; Watson *et al.* 2014). In addition, it has been suggested that coercive practices can contribute to an experience of the mental health system as punitive, unjust and harmful, which, in turn, can damage the establishment of therapeutic relationships, increase the time spent in hospital and dissuade people from further engagement with mental health services (Knowles *et al.* 2015; McLaughlin *et al.* 2016).

While the use of coercive practices is overwhelmingly identified as a negative experience, there is research to suggest that some people who have been subjected to them do come to perceive that those interventions were necessary to maintain their safety or the safety of others (Sibitz *et al.* 2011). However, while coercive practices are experienced differently by different people, and while the same individual can hold different views in relation to different instances of their use, a common theme that emerges from the available research is that there is a need for an improvement in the way in which those practices are employed. In particular, service users/survivors frequently question the extent to which a coercive intervention was necessary, the degree to which they received a clear rationale for its use, and the lack of concern, dignity and respect with which the measure was implemented (Sibitz *et al.* 2011; Looi *et al.* 2015).

ACTIVITY 6.5 RESEARCH

While the concept of epistemic injustice has recently been situated in the context of mental distress, psychiatry and health care (Crichton *et al.* 2016; Kidd & Carel 2017; Scrutton 2017), it was originally introduced by the philosopher Miranda Fricker (2007) to understand the injustices experienced by a variety of marginalised groups. In doing so, she maintains that epistemic injustice refers to the way in which a person can be treated unjustly in their capacity as someone who can possess and communicate knowledge. As she makes clear, 'This idea of being wronged in one's capacity as a knower constitutes my generic characterization of epistemic injustice' (Fricker 2008, p. 69).

In developing the notion of epistemic injustice, however, Fricker makes a distinction between two interrelated forms which she refers to as testimonial injustice and hermeneutical injustice. In testimonial injustice, a person's word or testimony – whether verbal or written – is understood by others as having minimal credibility owing to some form of prejudice or negative stereotype that is held about the person who gives the testimony. In contrast, hermeneutical injustice refers to the way in which a person's ability to make sense of their experience is disadvantaged by the existence of various restrictions that limit the opportunities that are available for a person to do so.

In the context of mental health services, testimonial injustice can occur when the experiences communicated by users/survivors are taken to be unreliable, inaccurate or irrelevant owing to various prejudices and negative stereotypes that are held about the character and capabilities of those who experience mental distress. In contrast, hermeneutical injustice can occur when the dominance of certain ways of understanding mental distress restrict the opportunities that service users/survivors have to make sense of their experience in their own terms and, where they attempt to do so, this meaning is subordinated to the meaning that is ascribed to that experience by others.

FURTHER READING

- **Beresford P** (2010) *A Straight Talking Introduction to Being a Mental Health Service User*. Ross-on-Wye: PCCS Books.

This book provides a comprehensive and accessible introduction to the service user/survivor movement and discusses its origins, its diverse concerns and objectives, as well as its possible future directions.

- **Chamberlin J** (1978) *On Our Own: Patient Controlled Alternatives to the Mental Health System*. New York, NY: Haworth Press.

Here you will find a foundational text for the service user/survivor movement that is concerned, among other things, with the development and delivery of user-controlled alternatives to existing mental health services.

- **LeFrançois BA, Menzies R & Reaume G** (eds) (2013) *Mad Matters: A Critical Reader in Canadian Mad Studies*. Toronto: Canadian Scholars' Press Inc.

With contributions from users/survivors, academics, practitioners and activists, this book displays the diverse theoretical and practical concerns that characterise the emerging and dynamic field of inquiry known as Mad Studies.

- **Russo J & Sweeney A** (eds) (2016) *Searching for a Rose Garden: Challenging Psychiatry, Fostering Mad Studies*. Monmouth: PCCS Books.

Primarily written by 'psychiatric survivors', this book critiques the ongoing dominance of certain approaches to mental distress and details the attempts of survivors to question, challenge and change those approaches.

USEFUL WEBSITES

- www.enusp.org

This is the website of the European Network for (ex)-Users and Survivors of Psychiatry, which is concerned with challenging discrimination against users/survivors and fighting for user-controlled alternatives to psychiatry.

- www.mindfreedom.org

Here you will find the website for MindFreedom International, which aims to protect the human rights of those who experience mental distress and to promote safe and humane forms of mental health care.

- www.nsun.org.uk

This is the website for the National Survivor User Network, an independent, service-user-led organisation which provides advice, support and information in order to influence mental health policy makers and service providers.

7

RECOVERY

CHAPTER AIMS

By the end of this chapter you will be able to:

- appraise the personal accounts of recovery;
- debate the co-option of recovery;
- evaluate the conditions that support recovery.

INTRODUCTION

👥 CASE STUDY

Mosi has been a mental health professional for over twenty years and during that time he has witnessed many changes in mental health care. As he reflects upon those changes with a colleague, he suggests that perhaps the most significant development has been an increased concern with recovery. Indeed, while this contemporary concern can be understood as being influenced by the personal accounts of those with experience of mental distress, the notion of recovery has now been widely adopted by the mental health system. As a consequence, there is an explicit requirement placed upon mental health professionals to become recovery-focused practitioners, and a variety of frameworks, initiatives and strategies have been introduced in order to support this development. Mosi therefore suggests that recovery is not an initiative that is comparable to previous changes that he has witnessed throughout his career. Rather, it has become a pervasive and powerful agenda that has profoundly influenced the manner in which, as a practitioner, he is now required to understand and respond to mental distress.

As highlighted by Mosi in the above case study, a concern with recovery has increasingly come to characterise contemporary mental health care. While this concern can be understood as having its origins within, and being profoundly influenced by, the accounts of recovery given by those with personal experience of mental distress, the notion of recovery has been widely adopted by mental health services. However, despite the recovery-focused reorientation of those services, and the requirement placed upon mental health professionals to become recovery-focused practitioners, a variety of critical issues surround the principles and practices that have come to be associated with the notion of recovery (Pilgrim & McCranie 2013; Slade *et al.* 2014; Beresford 2015). For example, there are critical considerations about the meaning of recovery and the way in which that notion, as it is formulated by those with personal experience of that process, has been adapted, distorted and ultimately subverted by the mental health system. In addition, there are critical discussions about the conditions that are necessary to support recovery and the manner in which the values, principles and practices associated with that notion can be reconciled with the range of objectives that mental health services are expected to meet. Moreover, there are provocative analyses about the extent to which recovery, by being adopted by the mental health system, has come to serve a variety of wider social, economic and political interests rather than empowering people who experience mental distress to explore and determine the character of their own recovery.

The purpose of this chapter is therefore to introduce you to a variety of critical issues surrounding recovery in contemporary mental health care. While recovery has been understood in a variety of ways, this chapter will begin by examining the manner in which it is often formulated by those with personal experience of that process. In doing so, it will not only consider the way in which recovery is commonly presented as a unique and individual journey, but it will also discuss how that journey is often concerned with reclaiming or creating a productive, fulfilling and meaningful life. This chapter will then critically consider the manner in which recovery, through being adopted by the mental health system, has been co-opted by and assimilated into that system. In particular, we shall examine how the recovery-focused reorientation of mental health services is said to have entailed, among other things, a theoretical and practical marginalisation of the way in which recovery is formulated by those who use mental health services. Finally, while acknowledging that the co-option of recovery by the mental health system should be a source of considerable concern, this chapter will propose that the personal accounts of recovery are an enduring testament to the fact that recovery is possible. In doing so, we shall examine how those accounts can be understood as a valuable resource by which to consider the conditions that are conducive to recovery and that enable mental health professionals to understand what they can do in their everyday practice to support a person's recovery.

THE PERSONAL ACCOUNTS OF RECOVERY

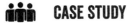 **CASE STUDY**

Following a diagnosis of schizophrenia in her early twenties, Ruth remembers the over-whelming sense of pessimism and hopelessness that she felt about her future. For many years after receiving this diagnosis she suggests that she effectively 'gave up' on herself and, during repeated mental health hospital admissions, became progressively more with-drawn, isolated and disenchanted with life. However, during one admission she remembers feeling profoundly angry and even outraged about the course her life was taking and began to develop a belief that it could and should be different. While Ruth finds it difficult to explain how and why this change occurred, she believes that this was when she began to challenge the pessimism that had dominated her life for so long and started to feel that she could reclaim a meaningful and fulfilling future. At that stage, she was unsure what form this future would take and how she was going to work towards it, but she suggests that this was the moment when she began the long and challenging journey that constituted her recovery.

Unlike many concepts in mental health care, contemporary notions about recovery have been profoundly influenced by the personal accounts of those with experience of mental distress (Chamberlin 1978; Deegan 1988; Coleman 1999). By reflecting upon that experience, and the insights that were obtained through confronting the challenges associated with it, those accounts often present recovery as a unique and personal journey (Unzicker 1989; O'Hagan 2014). In doing so, they not only highlight the difficulty of reconciling the experience of recovery with the theoretical principles and practices that have dominated mental health care, but they also maintain that it cannot adequately be described by using the language associated with traditional models of mental distress and the discourse of deficit that has characterised those models. However, while recovery is presented as a unique and individual journey, the personal accounts of that process typically emphasise the importance of hope, optimism and a belief that recovery is possible. Confronted with the variety of challenges that are associated with mental distress, recovery is presented as being characterised by a belief that those challenges can not only be endured but they can also be overcome. Indeed, in highlighting both the centrality of hope for recovery and the challenge of accommodating that quality within existing approaches to mental distress, Deegan (1988) proposes that 'All of the polemic and technology of psychiatry, psychology, social work, and science cannot account for this phenomenon of hope. But those of us who have recovered know that this grace is real. We lived it. It is our shared secret' (p. 14).

In the context of the recovery-focused reorientation of mental health care, the suggestion that recovery is possible may seem an unremarkable and insignificant claim. In order to understand its enduring significance, however, it is productive to contrast this claim with the pessimism that has traditionally been associated with mental distress. In so far as such distress has been understood as the manifestation of some form of individual and predominately biological 'disorder', 'disease' or 'illness', one of the enduring assumptions about such 'illnesses' is that they either deteriorate over time or, if they do not deteriorate, then they are likely to be persistent, recurring and require ongoing psychiatric intervention. While such pessimism has historically varied depending upon a range of factors, such as the specific psychiatric diagnosis under consideration, those who have used mental health services have highlighted how they either explicitly or implicitly received powerful messages from others to revise, and invariably to lower, the aspirations and expectations that they had previously held for their lives (Deegan 1996; Longden 2010). However, by giving prominence to hope and optimism, the personal accounts of those who have experience of recovery can be understood as presenting a radical challenge to such assumptions. In particular, by asserting that recovery is possible, those accounts resist enduring notions, both within and beyond the mental health system, about the supposedly chronic character of mental distress and the therapeutic pessimism that has been, and in some instances continues to be, associated with psychiatric diagnoses (King 2014).

─────── PRACTICE ISSUE: THERAPEUTIC PESSIMISM ───────

While the recent reorientation of mental health services towards recovery-focused practice has been influenced by the accounts of people who use those services, notions of recovery have intermittently been present throughout the history of mental health care. For example, it has been suggested that the origins of the contemporary concern with recovery can be traced back to the late 18th century and to the *traitement moral* associated with the work of the French physician Philippe Pinel at the Bicêtre and Salpêtrière institutions in Paris and the 'moral treatment' developed by the tea merchant and Quaker William Tuke at the Retreat in York (Davidson *et al.* 2010). Although their approaches had significant differences, Pinel and Tuke both rejected the hopelessness, repression and brutality that was characteristic of the asylums at the time, and maintained that, with humane treatment, psychological support and 'moral management', recovery was possible (Scull 2016).

Despite such historical instances, mental distress has commonly been associated with a pessimism about the possibility of recovery. While this has taken a variety of forms, it can be understood as being exemplified in the work of the 19th-century German psychiatrist Emil Kraepelin and his introduction of the diagnostic category *dementia praecox* – subsequently reformulated by the Swiss psychiatrist Eugen Bleuler as schizophrenia. Assumed to be the manifestation of some form of biological disorder, Kraepelin maintained that *dementia praecox*, was a condition characterised by an irreversible deterioration of the cognitive faculties. Rather than being based solely upon clinical observation, it has been suggested that this pessimism was influenced by the 19th-century **degeneration theory,** which, in sublimated form, is said to have had an enduring influence on assumptions about the possibility of recovery for those receiving a diagnosis of schizophrenia (Zubin *et al.* 1985; Blom & van Praag 2011).

By asserting the centrality of hope and optimism, and therefore challenging the pessimism that has been associated with mental distress, the personal accounts of those who have experience of recovery are resolutely focused on moving forward and the reclamation of a future. It is important to recognise, however, that this future is not presented in terms of the absence of mental distress and the removal of the sometimes complex, confusing and disturbing experiences that can be associated with that distress (Repper & Perkins 2012). Indeed, it has been suggested that recovery in the context of mental health care should be distinguished from that which has been referred to as 'clinical recovery', where this has been understood as the reduction and removal of the symptoms associated with various psychiatric diagnoses (Slade 2009; Roberts & Boardman 2013). While there is an acknowledgement that symptom reduction is desirable, the personal accounts of those with experience of recovery maintain that it is a journey that does not and should not refer to an endpoint or final destination that is characterised in terms of a 'cure', a return to 'previous levels of functioning' or seeking to somehow 'get back to normal'. Instead, recovery is presented as an on-going, episodic and non-liner process in which a person will encounter a variety of challenges and set-backs, including the recurrence, and even in some cases the continuation, of those complex and potentially disturbing experiences that can be associated with mental distress (Deegan 1993).

Rather than being understood in terms of symptom reduction, the hope and optimism that is characteristic of recovery is concerned with retrieving or creating a productive, fulfilling and meaningful life (Anthony 1993). While this endeavour may have common elements, what constitutes a meaningful life will be specific to each individual, and the personal accounts of recovery highlight the importance of being empowered to explore and discover what this means for each person (Gosling 2010). In doing so, those accounts maintain that this process can involve profound personal growth, development and transformation as an individual seeks to make sense of, come to terms with and then move beyond the event of mental distress and the various limitations that may have been, and that may continue to be, placed upon them by that distress (Houghton 1982). For example, a person may need to consider which of their attitudes, values and beliefs require revision, what relationships, attachments and associations they ought to maintain and what knowledge, skills and resources they must acquire in order to facilitate their recovery journey. Indeed, in so far as the experience of mental distress can alter an individual's identity, it has been suggested that recovery can even necessitate the development of a new sense of self as a person considers who they may need to become in order to accommodate the experience of mental distress into their lives, and, from the ground of that experience, nurture a new sense of direction, meaning and purpose (Deegan 1993; Roberts 2008).

─────── **CONCEPT SUMMARY: THE MEANING OF RECOVERY** ───────

Despite becoming increasingly prominent in mental health care, recovery is a complex and contested concept that has been formulated in a variety of ways. In seeking to provide a concise overview of the manner in which that notion has variously been understood, Pilgrim and McCranie (2013) identify four different meanings of recovery that, while conceptually distinguishable, may overlap in practice.

- **Recovery as a personal journey** is a prevalent formulation that is commonly expressed in the personal accounts of those who use mental health services. Understood as an individual process that is characterised by hope, courage and personal transformation, recovery is concerned with developing a meaningful life, not only in spite of, but sometimes precisely because of, the challenges associated with mental distress.
- **Recovery as a critique of services** is a powerful although less prevalent meaning that has been most closely associated with the service user/survivor movement. Against the pathologising and paternalistic approaches to mental distress that are said to characterise mental health services, recovery is understood as an alternative approach that promotes the self-determination and expertise of people who use those services.
- **Recovery as therapeutic optimism** is a formulation that opposes the therapeutic pessimism that has been associated with mental distress. While often presented as a belief in the possibility of recovering a meaningful life, it has also been understood as being synonymous with clinical recovery and referring to an optimism about the effectiveness of services to manage, reduce and even remove symptoms.
- **Recovery as a social model of disability** is a formulation that has been closely associated with some service user/survivor groups. Against understanding mental distress in terms of an individual dysfunction or deficit, recovery is concerned with facilitating social inclusion by challenging the stigma, discrimination and disabling social responses that those who use mental health services can experience from others.

In presenting recovery as an individual journey that is concerned with reclaiming or creating a meaningful life, the personal accounts of that process emphasise its difficulties, opportunities and wider dimensions. In doing so, they not only propose that profound personal transformation may be required in order to confront and move beyond the challenges that can arise as a consequence of the experiences or symptoms associated with mental distress; rather, they typically maintain that this can also involve recovering from the experience of the mental health system and the treatment that has been received from practitioners (May *et al.* 2015; O'Hagan 2016). For example, those who use mental health services often highlight the need to re-evaluate how their mental distress has been presented to them as the manifestation of some form of individual dysfunction or deficit, as well as the importance of reclaiming and redefining the experience of mental distress in their own terms. In addition, they also discuss how it has been necessary to recover from the various physiological and psychological consequences of treatment, such as the adverse effects of psychiatric drugs, as well as witnessing or being subject to a range of coercive practices that can occur in mental health settings, including seclusion, restraint and forced medication. Moreover, the personal accounts of recovery also emphasise how that process can involve confronting the negative stereotypes and stigma that are commonly associated with psychiatric diagnoses, and, in so far as a person comes to internalise that stigma, overcoming the sense of hopelessness, helplessness and isolation that this may produce.

Although recovery has been formulated as a personal journey, it is important to recognise that it is a journey which occurs within a broader social context. Indeed, the personal accounts of recovery are characteristically situated within this broader context and highlight the discrimination, prejudice and social exclusion that people who experience mental distress have to endure and seek to overcome (Leete 1989; Deegan 1992). While such discrimination can affect the lives of people in diverse ways, it can typically manifest as reduced employment, education and recreational opportunities; limited financial resources, insecure living arrangements and fewer supportive relationships; as well as a range of negative societal images, stereotypical assumptions and exclusionary beliefs about mental distress (Perkins & Repper 2013; Sayce 2016). Moreover, these multiple manifestations of discrimination can be compounded by a variety of wider social, economic and political determinants, such as the occurrence of economic recessions, local and national decisions on health and welfare expenditure, and the levels of wealth inequality throughout society more generally (Compton & Shim 2015). As a unique and personal journey, the challenges associated with recovery are therefore not confined to addressing the consequences of the symptoms that can be associated with mental distress or with the treatment that has been received from mental health services. Rather, it is a process that can involve the considerable challenge of confronting the multiple forms of discrimination that can obstruct the rights of people who experience mental distress and which can limit their opportunities to recover a productive, fulfilling and meaningful life.

ACTIVITY 7.1   CRITICAL THINKING

In seeking to address the stigma and discrimination surrounding mental distress, an enduring approach, routinely employed by anti-stigma campaigns, has been to promote the idea that such distress 'is an illness just like any other illness'. Rather than reducing stigma, however, there is evidence to suggest this approach may reinforce stereotypical assumptions about mental distress (Read *et al.* 2013; Malla *et al.* 2015).

For this activity think critically about the proposition that understanding mental distress as an illness like any other may contribute to the stigma and discrimination experienced by service users/survivors. As you do so, attempt to explain why that understanding of mental distress might perpetuate rather than reduce stereotypical assumptions and exclusionary beliefs about those who experience such distress.

An outline answer is provided at the end of the chapter.

THE CO-OPTION OF RECOVERY

 CASE STUDY

In their capacity as users of mental health services, Tamara and Jacob are discussing the effect that the contemporary concern with recovery has had upon those services and the mental health care that people receive. Jacob suggests that recovery has profoundly transformed how mental health professionals understand and respond to mental distress, and that, in recent years, it is probably the most important development in mental health care. While Tamara acknowledges that recovery has value, at least in how it is formulated by those with experience of mental distress, she has a number of concerns about the manner in which that notion has been adopted and adapted by the mental health system. However, Jacob replies that he simply cannot understand how anyone could have concerns about the recovery-focused reorientation of mental health services. In particular, he proposes that in contrast to the overwhelming pessimism and hopelessness that used to be associated with mental distress, the reorientation of mental health services towards recovery-focused practice, and the hope and optimism that it engenders, has unquestionably been a positive development.

As maintained by Jacob in the above case study, the recovery-focused reorientation of mental health services is often considered to be an unequivocally positive development in mental health care. Contrasted with the enduring pessimism and paternalism that has been associated with mental health services, recovery-focused practice is commonly understood as that which empowers people to consider, pursue and achieve their self-defined goals and aspirations. Indeed, it has been suggested that this characterisation of recovery has become so dominant in mental health care that raising any critical questions about the principles and practices associated with recovery can come to be seen as 'cynical' and 'mean-minded' (Beresford 2015). Despite its widespread adoption within mainstream mental health services, however, there has been sustained critical discussion, debate and dispute surrounding recovery, and this has been conducted variously by service users/survivors, mental health professionals and a range of academics and researchers affiliated with mental health care (Harper & Speed 2012; Slade *et al.* 2014; Williams 2016). While such discussions are diverse, multifaceted and employ a variety of theoretical perspectives, an overriding concern has been with the way in which the recovery-focused reorientation of mental health services has led to the co-option of recovery. In particular, there are ongoing critical considerations about the extent to which the mental health system, by adopting the notion of recovery, has adapted, distorted and ultimately subverted its meaning so that recovery-focused practice satisfies the objectives, requirements and demands of mental health services rather than the needs of the people who use those services.

Although it has been understood in a variety of ways, the co-option of recovery has commonly been presented in terms of a tension between personal recovery and clinical recovery (Slade 2009). In particular, it has been suggested that the mental health system has situated the notion of recovery within its dominant theoretical and therapeutic frameworks, which understand mental distress as the manifestation of some form of individual dysfunction or deficit. In this context, the notion of recovery has been associated with the treatment of these underlying deficits, and the reduction or removal of the symptoms that they supposedly produce, through the use of a variety of pharmacological and psychological means (Dillon 2011; Repper & Perkins 2012; Slade & Wallace 2017). As highlighted above, however, while the reduction of symptoms may be a desirable outcome, the personal accounts of those with experience of mental distress maintain that it is not a necessary condition for recovery. Rather than being understood as an end-point, destination or outcome that is defined in terms of a cure or the establishment of previous levels of functioning, those accounts maintain that recovery is an ongoing and non-linear process that is concerned with reclaiming or creating a productive, fulfilling and meaningful life. Therefore, despite the rhetoric of empowering people to pursue their self-defined goals, it has been suggested that the recovery-focused reorientation of mental health services has increasingly become associated with the professionally defined goals of symptom remission, relapse reduction and discharge from services.

PRACTICE ISSUE: RISK AND RECOVERY

One of the fundamental critical issues surrounding the adoption of a recovery-focused approach in mental health care is concerned with the extent to which it can be reconciled with the range of objectives that mental health services are expected to meet. In particular, it has been suggested that there exists a fundamental and recurring contradiction between the values, principles and practices that inform a recovery-focused approach to mental distress and the requirement placed upon mental health services to effectively regulate the range of risks that are commonly perceived to be associated with such distress (Pilgrim & McCranie 2013). For example, while recovery-focused practice is presented as being concerned with fostering hope, facilitating involvement and empowering those who use mental health services, the management of risk has often been associated with imposing restrictions, ensuring containment and asserting professional dominance.

While recognising the challenge in reconciling a recovery-focused approach to mental distress with the requirement placed upon mental health services to effectively regulate risk, it has been suggested that the two need not necessarily be mutually exclusive. Indeed, the personal accounts of recovery highlight that risk is not only fundamental to the exploration of how to manage and move beyond the event of mental distress but it can also be a valuable stimulus for the personal growth and development that is characteristic of recovery (Deegan 1996). In this context, it has been suggested that it is possible for mental health services to adopt a **positive risk-taking** approach to mental distress that, through the co-production of individual safety plans, supports a person's positive potential to manage risk and take control over their lives as they determine the character of their own recovery (Morgan 2013; Boardman & Roberts 2014).

In so far as it has come to be associated with clinical recovery, the manner in which recovery is formulated by those with personal experience of mental distress is said to have been progressively marginalised by the mental health system. Instead of being a unique qualitative process that involves the reclamation or creation of a meaningful life, where this is determined by the individual, recovery has come to be understood in terms of a set of quantifiable outcomes, such as symptom remission and relapse reduction, that can be monitored and measured by others. However, this reformulation of recovery not only marginalises an understanding of the unique character of the recovery process and its broader concerns with establishing a new sense of direction, meaning and purpose; rather, the co-option of recovery is also said to entail a theoretical and practical marginalisation of the wider social context in which recovery occurs. As highlighted above, despite presenting recovery as an individual journey, the personal accounts of that process often maintain that it is a journey which is situated within a wider social context. In particular, those accounts commonly highlight the way in which recovery involves enduring and seeking to overcome multiple manifestations of stigma, discrimination and social exclusion. However, by associating recovery with symptom reduction, it has been suggested that recovery-focused practice has increasingly come to be understood in terms of the provision of individualised interventions such as psychiatric drugs and psychotherapy rather than the development of strategies designed to address the multiple forms of discrimination which service users/survivors often confront (Perkins 2015).

While constituting a significant departure from how recovery is commonly presented by those with personal experience of mental distress, it has been suggested that the theoretical and practical marginalisation of the wider social context in which recovery occurs is politically expedient. Indeed, one of the central critical concerns about the recovery-focused reorientation of mental health services is the manner in which the reformulation of the notion of recovery has become allied to a variety of political interests (Braslow 2013; McWade 2016). In particular, it has been suggested that the association of recovery with clinical recovery enables political attention to be directed to the provision of comparatively inexpensive pharmacological and psychological interventions, rather than the more financially and politically demanding task of attempting to address the multiple forms of social injustice, inequality and discrimination which can obstruct a person's recovery. By marginalising the wider social context in which recovery occurs, the co-option of recovery by the mental health system is therefore said to be consistent with the interests of contemporary capitalist society and the political, economic and ideological commitment to reduce state intervention and public expenditure that is characteristic of neoliberalism. Indeed, in so far as recovery has also become associated with attempts to enhance the resilience of people to self-manage mental distress, as well as deal with a range of social adversities on their own, then there are concerns that recovery is being used as a 'neoliberal smokescreen' to cut mental health services, withdraw welfare benefits and indiscriminately drive service users/survivors into the labour market (Morrow 2013; Beresford 2015).

PRACTICE ISSUE: RESILIENCE AND RECOVERY

A complex and contested concept, the notion of resilience has variously been understood as an attribute, a process and an outcome that can be associated with individuals, organisations and even entire communities (Southwick *et al.* 2014). Despite such complexity, however, the notion of resilience is commonly presented in individualised terms as the ability of a person to positively respond to, or 'bounce back' and recover from, a range of adverse life events. Moreover, there has been increased interest, across a variety of areas, in facilitating the development of individual resilience through the use of various forms of psychological interventions and self-help strategies (Schiraldi 2017; Kain & Terrell 2018). In doing so, such psychological resilience is not only understood as an attribute that can prepare individuals to deal with adversity, and minimise the harm that it can produce, but it is also presented as a tool that can enable people to overcome and move beyond such adversity when it occurs (Southwick & Charney 2012).

While the attempt to facilitate the development of resilience is often understood as a productive intervention, there are critical concerns about its wider social and political implications. In particular, it has been suggested that the cultivation of psychological resilience serves to shift the responsibility to address the various forms of injustice, inequality and discrimination that exist within society away from governments, and instead places the onus on individuals to endure those social adversities (Harrison 2013; Diprose 2015). This relocation of responsibility is said to progressively undermine a sense of solidarity with others and diminish the likelihood of collective demands for political action. For example, rather than joining with others and looking outwards towards governments to address the challenges associated with insecure employment, economic recessions or wealth inequality, 'citizens are enjoined to look inward, gather their strengths, and be resilient' (Howell & Veronka 2012, pp. 4–5).

To raise concerns about the way in which recovery-focused practice has come to be understood in terms of the provision of individualised interventions and the facilitation of psychological resilience is not to disregard the value of such interventions. Rather, it is to maintain that a comprehensive approach to recovery, while acknowledging the role of individual interventions in supporting that process, ought to give at least equal consideration to the development of strategies designed to address the multiple challenges that characterise the social context in which recovery occurs (Perkins & Repper 2013; Sayce 2016). By marginalising this wider context, however, the co-option of recovery by the mental health system has led to an unduly individualised, predominately clinical and therefore fundamentally imbalanced understanding of recovery. Moreover, by becoming allied to a variety of political, economic and ideological interests, it has been suggested that this reformulation of the notion of recovery has come to acquire significant normative power such that recovery is progressively being transformed from a possibility into an imperative (Rose 2014; Edwards 2015). The recovery-focused reorientation of mental health services has therefore not merely become associated with the assumption that recovery is possible for everyone, irrespective of the form that a person's mental distress takes or the psychiatric diagnosis that they receive; rather, there are also critical concerns that a powerful expectation is further being placed upon people who use mental health services to engage with the recovery agenda and, significantly, to do so in ways determined by those services.

The requirement to engage with the recovery agenda, and the means used by mental health services to ensure that this requirement is met, can become manifest in a variety of ways. However, arguably the most contentious is the manner in which coercive practices such as seclusion, restraint and forced medication have been used within services that are supposedly recovery-focused, and, in particular, the way in which recovery has been presented as a rationale to justify those practices (Morgan & Felton 2015). While it has been argued that coercion is not opposed to recovery (Geller 2012), its use constitutes a profound departure from the values, principles and practices which those with personal experience of mental distress maintain are characteristic of the recovery process. Indeed, the personal accounts of recovery not only highlight the manner in which it is often necessary to recover from witnessing or being subject to a range of coercive practices. Rather, they also emphasise the importance of collaboration, self-determination and each individual being empowered to explore and pursue their own recovery path, as part of a unique and individual journey that is concerned with the reclamation or creation of a productive, fulfilling and meaningful life. Therefore, irrespective of other arguments that might be presented in order to justify coercive practices in mental health care, it has been suggested that the paternalism that is associated with the use of coercion cannot be reconciled with the values of choice and self-determination that are fundamental to the recovery process (Slade *et al.* 2014).

ACTIVITY 7.2   RESEARCH

While many service users/survivors value the emphasis placed upon recovery in mental health care, others are critical of what this has come to mean in practice. In particular, it has been suggested that although the notion of recovery is productive, the ways in which it has been adopted and adapted by mental health services has undermined the credibility that it had with the people who use those services (Beresford *et al.* 2016).

For this activity go to the website of Recovery in the Bin (www.recoveryinthebin.org), which is a service-user/survivor-led organisation that maintains a critical position in relation to recovery. As you explore the website, attempt to provide a concise overview of Recovery in the Bin's critique of recovery as well as a summary of the alternative approach to mental distress that it would like to see adopted.

An outline answer is provided at the end of the chapter.

SUPPORTING RECOVERY

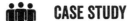 **CASE STUDY**

Although she has found it challenging, Ida has been conducting her own investigations into the critical issues that surround the co-option of recovery. While she had previously thought that the recovery-focused reorientation of mental health services was an unequivocally positive development, these investigations have led her to develop various concerns about how recovery has been adopted, adapted and implemented in the mental health setting in which she works. However, despite these concerns, she maintains that the personal accounts of those who have sought to overcome the challenges associated with mental distress have convinced her that the notion of recovery continues to have value. Indeed, she maintains that these personal accounts are a rich resource by which practitioners can understand the conditions that are conducive to recovery. Therefore, while she has developed a more sophisticated critical appreciation of the notion of recovery in mental health care, she continues to be committed to developing her ability to support the recovery of those who use mental health services.

As a consequence of concerns about the co-option of recovery by the mental health system, there are ongoing critical discussions about the significance, credibility and utility of that notion in contemporary mental health care. In particular, these discussions are centred around the extent to which the co-option of recovery can be resisted, and the productive elements of that notion retained, or whether recovery has become so distorted by the mental health system that it should now be abandoned (Trivedi 2010; Harper & Speed 2012; Beresford 2015). However, the personal accounts of those who have sought to confront and overcome the challenges associated with mental distress can be understood as an enduring testament to the fact that recovery is possible. Moreover, those accounts commonly highlight the way in which people are able to recover despite being situated within environments, and being subject to various attitudes and practices, that are not conducive to the recovery process. Therefore, while the reformulation of recovery by the mental health system, and the manner in which that notion has become allied to a variety of political, economic and ideological interests, should be a source of considerable concern, it should not be a source of despair. Indeed, the personal accounts of recovery not only attest to its possibility within the context of significant and seemingly insurmountable challenges, but, as Ida maintains in the above case study, they are also a valuable resource by which to understand what mental health professionals can do in their everyday practice to support a person's recovery.

Although a variety of frameworks, initiatives and strategies have been introduced in order to facilitate recovery, it is important to recognise that people cannot be made to recover. As a unique and personal process, recovery is a journey that is instigated by the individual, and, despite the prevalence of the recovery agenda throughout mental health services, a person cannot be willed, cajoled or coerced into undertaking that journey. However, while those who experience mental distress cannot be made to recover, it is possible to create conditions that are conducive to that process and which empower and support people throughout their recovery journey. In seeking to understand these conditions it is important to recognise that recovery occurs within the context of interpersonal relationships, and those who use mental health services maintain that the therapeutic quality of those relationships is fundamental to the recovery process (Simpson *et al.* 2016). As was highlighted in Chapter 5, relationships that have a positive, therapeutic effect upon a person's well-being are comprised of a variety of relational factors. However, the personal accounts of recovery consistently highlight that the condition that is central to that process is the presence of relationships that are characterised by hope, optimism and the belief that recovery is possible (Deegan 1988). In particular, those accounts emphasise the importance of others who believe in a person's potential to recover, and who, rather than overwhelming an individual with goals and future plans, skilfully communicates and nurtures this potential even when challenges, set-backs and crises occur.

———————— CONCEPT SUMMARY: THE CHIME FRAMEWORK ————————

The personal accounts of recovery highlight a variety of factors and conditions which are conducive to the recovery process. In providing a concise overview of these factors, Leamy *et al.* (2011) identify five 'recovery processes' – represented by the acronym CHIME – that form a framework by which to consider the conditions and structure interventions that support recovery.

- **Connectedness** refers to having contact with others and the importance of supportive relationships with family and friends, health care professionals and those who have experience of mental distress. In addition to a sense of belonging among others in the immediate environment, it also refers to feeling valued as a member of society.
- **Hope** and optimism emphasise the importance of believing that recovery is possible and having hope-inspiring relationships that nurture this belief, even when challenges and apparent set-backs occur. In maintaining hope about moving beyond the event of mental distress, it also highlights the importance of having goals, aspirations and dreams.
- **Identity** refers to that endeavour whereby a person seeks to reclaim their previous identity or develop a new identity that accommodates the experience of mental distress within their lives. In doing so, it highlights the importance of not being defined by psychiatric diagnoses and overcoming the stigma associated with those diagnoses.
- **Meaning** and purpose involve attempting to make sense of the experience of mental distress and reclaiming or creating a productive, fulfilling and meaningful life. While this can imply the development of an overarching sense of life's purpose, it also involves participation in meaningful activities, occupations and social roles.
- **Empowerment** refers to the control that a person has over the recovery process, and their life in general, and the extent to which they are involved in decisions about things which affect them. To aid this process, the importance of providing information and support to enhance a person's strengths, resources and potential is highlighted.

While establishing hope-inspiring relationships with people who experience mental distress is fundamental to the facilitation of recovery, it is necessary for this hope to be accompanied by action. However, although there are a variety of initiatives that have been designed to guide recovery-focused practice – such as the **Wellness Recovery Action Plan** (Copeland 1997) and the **Recovery Star** (McKeith & Burns 2011) – these should not be used in a prescriptive manner. While such initiatives can be productive in supporting recovery, there is no formula for this process. Rather, the personal accounts of recovery emphasise the importance of individuals being empowered to determine the character of their own recovery, and, in order to support this, the establishment of relationships and environments in which people are given choices and are permitted to make decisions. In seeking to promote such self-determination, the focus should not simply be on the provision of small, routine and everyday choices. Rather, the personal accounts of those with experience of recovery maintain the importance of formulating their own understanding of what may have contributed to the emergence and maintenance of mental distress, and, in doing so, reclaiming and redefining that experience in their own terms. In addition, those accounts also emphasise the necessity of having choices about what interventions may support recovery and, for example, being meaningfully involved in decisions about the use of psychiatric drugs. Moreover, the personal accounts of recovery also highlight the need for opportunities to explore which activities, occupations and social roles may enable a person to develop a new sense of direction and meaning in their lives and thereby move beyond the event of mental distress (Houghton 1982; Deegan & Drake 2006; Longden 2010).

In seeking to empower people to determine the character of their own recovery then it is necessary to adopt an approach that fosters the strengths, resources and potential of those who experience mental distress. In contrast to those approaches that have dominated mental health care, a strengths-based approach is not focused upon determining what deficits, limitations or weaknesses a person has. Rather, it is concerned with establishing collaborative relationships with those who use mental health services in order to identify the personal and environmental resources that they already possesses, and the resources that they may need to acquire in order to explore and pursue their own recovery path (Rapp & Goscha 2012). However, such an approach requires a recognition of, and a commitment to address, the imbalances in power that exist between those who use mental health services and those who provide such services. In presenting a concise summary of the transformation in values, attitudes and practices that such a shift in power necessitates, Perkins (2015) has proposed that practitioners need to move from being 'on top' to being 'on tap' (p. 40). That is, in seeking to promote the self-determination of those who experience mental distress, practitioners can no longer retain their traditional, paternalistic role of deciding how best to understand and respond to that distress. Rather, the knowledge, skills and experience of mental health professionals need to be positioned as a valuable and readily available resource that those who use mental health services can draw upon when required in order to explore and pursue a form of recovery that is best suited to their personal requirements (O'Hagan 2007).

ACTIVITY 7.3   RESEARCH

Originating in the Western part of Finnish Lapland, **open dialogue** is an approach to mental distress that is gaining increased attention around the world. This is not only because of its reported effectiveness, but also because of its consistency with recovery-focused principles and practices (Lakeman 2014; Seikkula 2015).

For this activity conduct your own investigations into open dialogue and provide a concise summary of this approach. As you do so, attempt to determine what are its characteristic features and the manner in which open dialogue can be understood as being different from established approaches to mental distress.

An outline answer is provided at the end of the chapter.

While emphasising the importance of being empowered to determine the character of their own recovery, the personal accounts of this process also repeatedly highlight the social context in which it occurs. In seeking to support recovery in this wider context, it has been suggested that the concern has typically been to reduce or remove the symptoms associated with a person's experience of mental distress while fostering their personal resources and resilience so that they are better able to 'cope with' and 'fit into' mainstream society (Perkins & Repper 2013). However, in seeking to situate and support recovery in its wider social context, the goal should not be to accommodate people to the requirements of society and, in doing so, leave unchallenged the various forms of injustice, inequality and discrimination that people who experience mental distress often confront. Rather, a comprehensive approach to recovery ought to be concerned with the development of strategies that are designed to address the challenges that characterise the social context in which recovery occurs and which can obstruct the reclamation or creation of a productive, fulfilling and meaningful life. Indeed, in expressing the need for recovery to become allied to a concern with social reform, Deegan (1996) memorably declares that 'The goal of recovery is not to get mainstreamed. We don't want to be mainstreamed. We say let the mainstream become a wide stream that has room for all of us and leaves no one stranded on the fringes' (p. 92).

The attempt to address the range of social adversities that can obstruct recovery is a prodigious task that requires the development and implementation of progressive social, economic and political strategies at both the local and national level. It has been suggested, however, that mental health professionals can engage in a variety of activities as part of their routine practice in order to promote the social inclusion of those who experience mental distress and their participation in society as citizens who have a right to the same opportunities that are afforded to other members of society (Perkins & Repper 2013; Sayce 2016). For example, practitioners can actively help those who use mental health services to identify and participate in a range of social, economic and leisure activities, and, in doing so, promote the type of interaction with other members of the community that challenges stigma, prejudice and discrimination. In addition, mental health professionals can use their position and influence to counter negative stereotypes and exclusionary beliefs about mental distress, and, in contrast to the idea that such distress 'is an illness just like any other', promote the strengths, resources and potential of those who use mental health services. Moreover, in seeking to support recovery in its wider social context, it has been suggested that practitioners should adopt a human-rights-based approach to mental health, which not only informs people about their legal rights as citizens but also provides support in seeking redress when the rights of those who experience mental distress have been breached.

CONCEPT SUMMARY: THE PANEL PRINCIPLES

A human-rights-based approach to mental health places various requirements on those involved in the provision of mental health care. In order to consider these requirements, five principles have been identified – represented by the acronym PANEL – which can be used to structure interventions that support the human rights of those who experience mental distress (SHRC 2016).

- **Participation** refers to the need to ensure people are meaningfully involved in the decisions which affect their lives. Also highlighted is the importance of providing those who experience mental distress with sufficient information and support to actively participate in decision-making processes.
- **Accountability** involves monitoring the human rights of those who use mental health services. It requires those services to have effective policies and procedures to uphold people's rights and to ensure that any breaches of those rights are recognised and redressed as soon as possible.
- **Non-discrimination** and equality refer to the identification and removal of all forms of discrimination. In addition, the importance of ensuring that people who experience mental distress have access to the same range of opportunities as other members of society is emphasised.
- **Empowerment** involves enabling people who use mental health services to understand and claim their rights. While it highlights the importance of providing information about human rights in an accessible form, it also requires that people have the necessary support to exercise those rights.
- **Legality** refers to a recognition that the human rights of those who experience mental distress are protected by national and international law. Thus, there is an emphasis on the importance of using this legal framework to monitor and maintain the full range of rights that people possess.

CHAPTER SUMMARY

This chapter has examined a variety of critical issues surrounding recovery in contemporary mental health care. While recovery has been understood in a variety of ways, this chapter has examined the manner in which it is often formulated by those with personal experience of that process. In doing so, it has not only considered the way in which recovery is commonly presented as a unique and individual journey, but it has also discussed how that journey is often concerned with reclaiming or creating a productive, fulfilling and meaningful life. Moreover, this chapter has critically considered the manner in which recovery, through being adopted by the mental health system, has been co-opted by and assimilated into that system. In particular, it has examined how the recovery-focused reorientation of mental health services is said to have entailed, among other things, a theoretical and practical marginalisation of the way in which recovery is formulated by those who use mental health services. Finally, while acknowledging that the co-option of recovery by the mental health system should be a source of considerable concern, this chapter has proposed that the personal accounts of recovery are an enduring testament to the fact that recovery is possible. In doing so, it has examined how those accounts can be understood as a valuable resource by which to consider the conditions that are conducive to recovery and that enable mental health professionals to understand what they can do in their everyday practice to support a person's recovery.

ACTIVITIES: BRIEF OUTLINE ANSWERS

ACTIVITY 7.1 CRITICAL THINKING

The typical rationale for promoting the idea that mental distress is an illness like any other is that if people who experience such distress are viewed as having an illness then others will respond, as people commonly do with medical illnesses, by displaying care and compassion. However, critical examination of this approach suggests that understanding mental distress as a medical issue is not only ineffective in reducing stigma and discrimination but may also worsen stereotypical assumptions and exclusionary beliefs about those who experience such distress (Read *et al.* 2013; Malla *et al.* 2015). In particular, the evidence indicates that if a person's mental distress is understood as a manifestation of some form of biological dysfunction, then that person is also more likely to be perceived by others as having limited control over their thoughts, feelings and behaviour. This perception can not only reinforce concerns about the supposedly chronic character of 'mental illness', but may also perpetuate fears about the unpredictability and dangerousness of those with such 'illnesses'. Therefore, rather than reducing stigma and discrimination, a biological understanding of mental distress can perpetuate prejudicial assumptions about such distress and increase a desire within others to maintain a high degree of social distance from those who use mental health services (Read *et al.* 2006; Schomerus *et al.* 2012).

ACTIVITY 7.2 RESEARCH

Recovery in the Bin's critique of recovery is multifaceted and expressed through various means, including its '20 Key Principles' and its development of the 'UnRecovery Star'. However, it proposes that recovery has become allied to the political interests of neoliberalism and this development has marginalised attempts to understand and respond to the challenges that characterise the social context in which people's lives are lived. Moreover, it maintains that recovery has been reformulated by mental health services in terms of a set of narrowly defined, quantifiable outcomes and is critical of the way in which this seeks to standardise an inherently individual and unique process. In addition, it is opposed to pressure being placed upon those who use mental health services to engage with the recovery agenda and rejects recovery being employed as a rationale for the use of any form of coercion.

While it is critical of what the recovery-focused reorientation of mental health services has come to mean in practice, Recovery in the Bin maintains that certain values associated with recovery, such as autonomy and self-determination, do have worth. However, it proposes that attempts to facilitate the autonomy and self-determination of those who experience mental distress must be situated within a wider social context. In particular, Recovery in the Bin calls for the adoption of a social model of mental distress to ensure greater recognition of the social determinants that can not only contribute to the emergence of mental distress but can also obstruct attempts to manage that distress. In doing so, it demands the development and implementation of comprehensive social, economic and political strategies to address these social determinants and thereby create environments that are more conducive to people's well-being.

ACTIVITY 7.3 RESEARCH

While open dialogue refers to a set of principles that can guide the provision of mental health services, it also refers to an intervention that can be used irrespective of the particular form that a person's mental distress takes or the psychiatric diagnosis that they receive (Seikkula 2015). In its broadest sense, open dialogue is an approach to mental health care, commonly employed to respond to severe mental health crisis situations, that seeks to elicit the resources of a person experiencing mental distress and those of their family and wider social support network. The basic forum for this approach is the treatment meeting, which includes the person, their support network and a range of mental health practitioners and other relevant agency members. Typically, this meeting occurs within the person's home within 24 hours of the mental health services being contacted, in order to commence the intervention as soon as possible in the context of the person's everyday environment and thereby reduce the likelihood of hospital admission.

What distinguishes these meetings from traditional interventions, however, is the emphasis placed on facilitating an open dialogue among all participants. In this way mental health professionals resist making theoretical and therapeutic assumptions about the situation, so that, rather than reaching premature treatment decisions, there is a focus on the development of a communal understanding of the situation in a shared language. Therefore, in contrast to those dysfunction- or illness-orientated approaches to mental distress that seek to reduce or remove symptoms, primarily through the use of psychiatric drugs, open dialogue is concerned with eliciting the resources of the person and their family in order to make sense of and move beyond the crisis. While psychiatric drugs are considered as a treatment option if discussed and decided on by all participants, they are generally thought to obstruct attempts to promote a person's own resources, self-determination and participation in the process that characterises open dialogue.

FURTHER READING

- **Pilgrim D & McCranie A** (2013) *Recovery and Mental Health: A Critical Sociological Account.* Basingstoke: Palgrave Macmillan.

An examination of recovery from a critical sociological perspective which includes an account of the different meanings of that notion and the manner in which recovery has been adopted by mental health services.

- **Rapp CA & Goscha RJ** (2012) *The Strengths Model: A Recovery-Orientated Approach to Mental Health Services,* 3rd edition. New York, NY: Oxford University Press.

In contrast to the dominance of a deficit-based approach in mental health care, this book details how to identify and support the strengths, resources and potential of those who experience mental distress.

- **Repper J & Perkins R** (2003) *Social Inclusion and Recovery: A Model for Mental Health Practice.* London: Ballière Tindall.

By drawing upon the personal accounts of those with experience of mental distress, this book provides a comprehensive account of supporting the process of recovery in the context of social inclusion.

- **Sayce L** (2016) *From Psychiatric Patient to Citizen Revisited.* London: Palgrave.

An examination of the discrimination that those who use mental health services often confront, including, in the context of a human-rights-based approach, a critical discussion of how that discrimination can be addressed.

USEFUL WEBSITES

- www.copelandcenter.com

This is the website for the Copeland Center for Wellness and Recovery, which provides a range of information and resources about supporting recovery by using the Wellness Recovery Action Plan (WRAP).

- www.igotbetter.org

In seeking to challenge the pessimism and hopelessness that has traditionally been associated with mental distress, this website provides a collection of videos and written stories about hope, recovery and mental well-being.

GLOSSARY

Acculturation: the process of change that occurs when a person or group from one culture encounters a person or group from other cultures.

Anti-psychiatry movement: the group of thinkers writing in the 1960s and 1970s who challenged the theoretical principles and practice of psychiatry.

Assumptions: ideas and beliefs that are assumed to be the case and, often without our explicit awareness, influence how we think, feel and act.

Autoethnography: a form of writing in which personal experience is analysed to illustrate wider cultural, social and political meanings associated with that experience.

Biomarker: a measurable biological characteristic that can mark or indicate the presence of a disease or pathological process.

Conscientisation: the process of gaining a critical awareness of the wider social, political and economic factors that are influencing one's life.

Construct: in the context of the voice-hearing experience, a collaborative interpretation of the possible significance and meaning of that experience.

Co-option: a process by which something is taken over by, and assimilated into, a larger or more established entity.

Critical psychiatry movement: a group of contemporary thinkers concerned with challenging, and seeking alternatives to, the technological model of mental distress.

Degeneration theory: a discredited 19th-century theory concerned with the supposed hereditary physical, mental and moral decline of human civilisation.

Developmental neuroscience: a field of inquiry that is concerned with the development of the nervous system.

Disabled people's movement: a global movement that seeks to secure rights, freedoms and equal opportunities for disabled people.

Discontinuation effect: a deterioration in well-being that arises as a consequence of the cessation or discontinuation of a drug.

Discourse of deficit: a body of knowledge, with associated terms and practices, in which notions of deficiency, dysfunction or disorder predominate.

Discrimination: the practice of treating a person or people less favourably because they possess, or are perceived as possessing, a particular characteristic.

Disease-centred model: the theory that psychiatric drugs work by correcting the biological dysfunctions that are claimed to be associated with mental distress.

Distal social determinants: the social factors associated with mental distress that exert their influence 'from a distance' and in an indirect, delayed manner.

Dodo bird verdict: A phrase used in relation to the claim that different psychotherapies produce roughly equivalent outcomes. It originates from the pronouncement of the dodo bird in Lewis Caroll's *Alice's Adventures in Wonderland*, who, after attempting to judge the outcome of a disorganised race between a variety of participants, reaches the verdict that 'everybody has won and all must have prizes'.

Drapetomania: the supposed 'disease of the mind', proposed by the 19th-century physician Samuel A Cartwright, that caused slaves to flee from their slavery.

Drug-centred model: the theory that psychiatric drugs cause a range of altered mental and physical states that can have negative and positive effects upon mental distress.

Dysphoria: a profound state of discomfort, dissatisfaction, unhappiness or frustration.

Epigenetics: a field of inquiry into the mechanisms by which factors beyond a person's genes, such as environmental stimuli, can influence the activity of those genes.

Epistemic injustice: a condition in which a person's opportunity to make sense of and communicate their experience is unjustly restricted.

Ex juvantibus: a form of reasoning in which one draws conclusions about the cause of a disease based upon the response of that disease to a particular treatment.

Extrapyramidal effects: a group of adverse effects produced by antipsychotic drugs, including acute dystonia, akathisia, Parkinsonism and tardive dyskinesia.

Genome: an organism's complete set of genetic material that contains all of the information required to build and maintain that organism.

Gross domestic product: the monetary value of all the goods and services produced by a country in a specific time period.

High expressed emotion: the hostility, over-involvement and criticism that can be expressed towards a family member who has been given a psychiatric diagnosis.

Hysteria: a supposed mental disorder, almost exclusively attributed to women, whose symptoms included nervousness, fainting, irritability and sexual desire.

Institutional racism: the perpetuation of negative attitudes and unequal treatment by an institution towards a person or people on the basis of their race.

Mad Studies: a field of inquiry and project of political engagement that is focused upon, and primarily conducted by, those with experiences of mental distress.

Microaggressions: the subtle, brief and casual comments and behaviours that demean, dismiss or humiliate people from marginalised groups.

Movement for global mental health: a coalition that seeks to improve the provision of mental health care in poorer, under-resourced countries.

Negative symptoms: the symptoms associated with a diagnosis of schizophrenia, such as apathy and lethargy, in which prior features of a person's experience are removed.

Neoliberalism: a political and economic ideology that prioritises individual self-reliance, competitive self-interest and free-market capitalism.

Normative assumptions: the assumptions that reflect the norms, values and beliefs about what is appropriate, acceptable or desirable.

Open dialogue: a social-network approach to mental distress that prioritises open discussion and full participation to make sense of and move beyond that distress.

Paradigm: a collection of assumptions, concepts and theories that form a framework by which to understand the world or an aspect of the world.

Placebo: an inactive substance that is administered to a person who believes that it is a genuine medicine with active ingredients.

Polypharmacy: the practice of prescribing multiple medications (commonly understood as four or more) to the same individual.

Positive risk-taking: a collaborative approach to risk management that promotes a person's potential to manage that risk as they pursue their stated priorities.

Positive symptoms: the symptoms associated with a diagnosis of schizophrenia, such as hallucinations and delusions, in which features are added to a person's experience.

Proximal social determinants: the social factors associated with mental distress that exert their influence 'from a close proximity' and in a direct, immediate manner.

Psychoactive substance: a chemical substance that acts upon the central nervous system to produce changes in perception, mood, consciousness or behaviour.

Qualitative research methodologies: research approaches (such as phenomenology, grounded theory, ethnography and case studies) that investigate people's experiences and the quality of those experiences.

Quantitative research methodologies: research approaches (such as randomised controlled trials, cohort studies, case-control studies and cross-sectional studies) that are adopted to obtain quantifiable data.

Randomised controlled trial: a research experiment in which participants are randomly assigned to receive one of two (or more) treatment interventions to determine the usefulness of those interventions.

Recovery Star: a recovery tool that identifies 10 dimensions of recovery and, for each dimension, a five-stage 'ladder of change' from 'stuck' to 'self-reliance'.

Serotonin syndrome: a drug-induced reaction associated with an excess of serotonin and characterised by various features including tremor, anxiety and restlessness.

Sick role: relating to the set of beliefs, behaviours and expectations associated with being 'sick' that are placed upon someone or that an individual may adopt.

Signs: the physical indications of the potential presence of a disease or disorder that can be detected by a variety of medical measures and technologies.

Soteria: relating to a psychiatric drug-free and minimum medication approach to mental distress in a non-medical community setting.

Stigma: a characteristic that is judged to be unwanted, and the disapproval of a person because they possess, or are perceived as possessing, this characteristic.

Stress-vulnerability: the notion that mental distress arises as a consequence of an interaction between the stress and challenging life events to which a person is subject, and that person's inherited or acquired vulnerabilities to such distress.

Symptoms: the subjective experiences and feelings about the potential presence of a disease or disorder that a person may report to health care professionals.

Technological model of mental distress: an approach in which mental distress is understood in predominately individualistic terms and responded to by using a variety of technical means.

Tokenistic: to meet a requirement in a minimal and superficial way that is nevertheless designed to give the appearance of genuine commitment.

Victim blaming: holding individuals responsible for the problems they experience, often by failing to consider the role of wider social factors in the emergence and maintenance of those problems.

Wellness Recovery Action Plan (WRAP): a recovery tool that supports a person to identify factors which maintain their mental well-being and deal with crises.

Whig histories: accounts of history that characterise the past in terms of a continuous development towards greater levels of social, political and cultural progress.

REFERENCES

Allen J, Balfour R, Bell R & Marmot M (2014) Social determinants of mental health. *International Review of Psychiatry*, 26(4): 392–407.

Al-Shawi HH (2011) *Reconstructing Subjects: A Philosophical Critique of Psychotherapy*. Amsterdam: Rodopi.

Anthony WA (1993) Recovery from mental illness: the guiding vision of the mental health service system in the 1990s. *Psychosocial Rehabilitation Journal*, 16(4): 11–23.

APA (American Psychiatric Association) (2013) *Diagnostic and Statistical Manual of Mental Disorders*, 5th edition (DSM-5). Washington, DC: American Psychiatric Association.

Arnstein SR (1969) A ladder of citizen participation. *Journal of the American Institute of Planners*, 35(4): 216–224.

Barker-Collo S & Read J (2003) Models of response to childhood sexual abuse: their implications for treatment. *Trauma, Violence & Abuse*, 4(2): 95–111.

Barlow DH (2010) Negative effects from psychological treatments: a perspective. *American Psychologist*, 65(1): 13–20.

Barnes TR (1989) A rating scale for drug-induced akathisia. *British Journal of Psychiatry*, 154(5): 672–676.

Barnes TRE (2011) Evidence-based guidelines for the pharmacological treatment of schizophrenia: recommendations from the British Association for Psychopharmacology. *Journal of Psychopharmacology*, 25(5): 567–620.

Barth J, Munder T, Gerger H ... Cuijpers P (2013) Comparative efficacy of seven psychotherapeutic interventions for patients with depression: a network meta-analysis. *PLoS Medicine*, 10(5): e1001454.

Beavan V, Read J & Cartwright C (2011) The prevalence of voice-hearers in the general population: a literature review. *Journal of Mental Health*, 20(3): 281–292.

Beck AT (1979) *Cognitive Therapy and the Emotional Disorders*. New York, NY: Penguin.

Bee P, Price O, Baker J & Lovell K (2015) Systematic synthesis of barriers and facilitators to service user-led care planning. *The British Journal of Psychiatry*, 207(2): 104–114.

Bentall RP (2004) *Madness Explained: Psychosis and Human Nature*. London: Penguin.

Bentall RP (2010) *Doctoring the Mind: Why Psychiatric Treatments Fail*. London: Penguin.

Bentall RP, de Sousa P, Varese F ... Read J (2014) From adversity to psychosis: pathways and mechanisms from specific adversities to specific symptoms. *Social Psychiatry and Psychiatric Epidemiology*, 49(7): 1011–1022.

Ben-Zeev D, Young MA & Corrigan PW (2010) DSM-V and the stigma of mental illness. *Journal of Mental Health*, 19(4): 318–327.

Beresford P (2010) *A Straight Talking Introduction to Being a Mental Health Service User*. Ross-on-Wye: PCCS Books.

Beresford P (2013) *Beyond the Usual Suspects: Towards Inclusive User Involvement*. London: Shaping Our Lives.

Beresford P (2015) From 'recovery' to reclaiming madness. *Clinical Psychology Forum*, 268: 16–20.

Beresford P (2016) The role of survivor knowledge in creating alternatives to psychiatry. In Russo J & Sweeney A (eds) *Searching for a Rose Garden: Challenging Psychiatry, Fostering Mad Studies*. Monmouth: PCCS Books, pp. 25–34.

Beresford P, Perring R, Nettle M & Wallcraft J (2016) *From Mental Illness to a Social Model of Madness and Distress*. London: Shaping Our Lives.

Berk M & Parker G (2009) The elephant on the couch: side-effects of psychotherapy. *Australian and New Zealand Journal of Psychiatry*, 43(9): 787–794.

Bjornestad J, Davidson L, Joa I ... Bronnick K (2017) Antipsychotic treatment: experiences of fully recovered service users. *Journal of Mental Health*, 26(3): 264–270.

Blom JD & van Praag HM (2011) Schizophrenia: it's broken and it can't be fixed. A conceptual analysis at the centenary of Bleuler's *Dementia praecox oder Gruppe der Schizophrenien*. *Israel Journal of Psychiatry and Related Sciences*, 48(4): 240–248.

Bloom BS, Engelhart MD, Furst EJ ... Krathwohl DR (1956) *Taxonomy of Educational Objectives: The Classification of Educational Goals. Handbook I: Cognitive Domain*. New York, NY: David McKay Company.

Bloom SL & Farragher B (2013) *Restoring Sanctuary: A New Operating System for Trauma-Informed Systems of Care*. New York, NY: Oxford University Press.

Boardman J & Roberts G (2014) *Risk, Safety and Recovery*. London: Centre for Mental Health and Mental Health Network, NHS Confederation.

Bola JR & Mosher LR (2003) Treatment of acute psychosis without neuroleptics: two-year outcomes from the Soteria project. *Journal of Nervous and Mental Disease*, 191(4): 219–229.

Bostock J, Noble V & Winter R (2012) Promoting community resources. In Newnes C, Holmes G & Dunn C (eds) *This is Madness: A Critical Look at Psychiatry and the Future of Mental Health Services*. Ross-on-Wye: PCCS Books, pp. 241–251.

Bourdieu P (1992) *Language and Symbolic Power*. Cambridge: Polity Press.

Bowie C, McLeod J & McLeod J (2016) 'It was almost like the opposite of what I needed': a qualitative exploration of client experiences of unhelpful therapy. *Counselling and Psychotherapy Research*, 16(2): 79–87.

Bowlby J (1969) *Attachment and Loss. Volume 1: Attachment*. New York, NY: Basic Books.

Boyle M (2011) Making the world go away, and how psychology and psychiatry benefit. In Rapley M, Moncrieff J & Dillon J (eds) *De-Medicalising Misery: Psychiatry, Psychology and the Human Condition*. Basingstoke: Palgrave Macmillan, pp. 27–43.

Boyle M (2012) Diagnosis. In Newnes C, Holmes G & Dunn C (eds) *This is Madness: A Critical Look at Psychiatry and the Future of Mental Health Services*. Ross-on-Wye: PCCS Books, pp. 75–90.

Boyle M (2015) The persistence of medicalisation: is the presentation of alternatives part of the problem? In Coles S, Keenan S & Diamond B (eds) *Madness Contested: Power and Practice*. Monmouth: PCCS Books, pp. 3–22.

Bracken P & Thomas P (2001) Postpsychiatry: a new direction for mental health. *British Medical Journal*, 322: 724–727.

Bracken P, Thomas P, Timimi S ... Yeomans D (2012) Psychiatry beyond the current paradigm. *The British Journal of Psychiatry*, 201(6): 430–434.

Braslow JT (2013) The manufacture of recovery. *Annual Review of Clinical Psychology*, 9: 781–809.

Breggin PR (1993) *Toxic Psychiatry*. London: Fontana.

Breggin PR (2006) Intoxication anosognosia: the spellbinding effect of psychiatric drugs. *Ethical Human Psychology and Psychiatry*, 8(3): 201–215.

Breggin PR (2013) *Psychiatric Drug Withdrawal: A Guide for Prescribers, Therapists, Patients, and their Families*. New York, NY: Springer.

Britten N, Riley R & Morgan M (2010) Resisting psychotropic medicines: a synthesis of qualitative studies of medicine-taking. *Advances in Psychiatric Treatment*, 16(3): 207–218.

Bronfenbrenner U (1979) *The Ecology of Human Development: Experiments by Nature and Design*. Cambridge, MA: Harvard University Press.

Brookfield SD (2001) *Developing Critical Thinkers: Challenging Adults to Explore Alternative Ways of Thinking and Acting*. Milton Keynes: Open University Press.

Brown C & Stansy P (2016) Peer workers in the mental health system: a transformative or collusive experiment. In Russo J & Sweeney A (eds) *Searching for a Rose Garden: Challenging Psychiatry, Fostering Mad Studies*. Monmouth: PCCS Books, pp. 183–191.

Busfield J (2011) *Mental Illness*. Cambridge: Polity Press.

Busfield J (2014) Transforming misery into sickness: the genealogy of depression in the Diagnostic and Statistical Manual. In Speed E, Moncrieff J & Rapley M (eds) *De-Medicalising Misery II: Society, Politics and the Mental Health Industry*. Basingstoke: Palgrave Macmillan, pp. 154–173.

Busfield J (2015) The pharmaceutical industry and mental disorder. In Coles S, Keenan S & Diamond B (eds) *Madness Contested: Power and Practice*. Monmouth: PCCS Books, pp. 90–110.

Butler G (1998) Clinical formulation. In Bellack AS & Hersen M (eds) *Comprehensive Clinical Psychology*. Oxford: Pergamon, pp. 1–24.

Calton T, Ferriter M, Huband N & Spandler H (2008) A systematic review of the Soteria paradigm for the treatment of people diagnosed with schizophrenia. *Schizophrenia Bulletin*, 34(1): 181–192.

Campbell P (2012) The service user/survivor movement. In Newnes C, Holmes G & Dunn C (eds) *This is Madness: A Critical Look at Psychiatry and the Future of Mental Health Services*. Ross-on-Wye: PCCS Books, pp. 195–209.

Campbell P (2013) Service users/survivors and mental health services. In Cromby J, Harper D & Reavey P (eds) *Psychology, Mental Health and Distress*. Basingstoke: Palgrave Macmillan, pp. 139–151.

Carr S & Patel M (2016) *Practical Guide: Progressing Transformative Co-production in Mental Health*. Bath: National Development Team for Inclusion.

Castonguay LG & Beutler LE (eds) (2006) *Principles of Therapeutic Change that Work*. New York, NY: Oxford University Press.

Castonguay LG & Hill CE (eds) (2007) *Insight in Psychotherapy*. Washington, DC: American Psychological Association.

Chamberlin J (1978) *On Our Own: Patient-Controlled Alternatives to the Mental Health System*. New York, NY: Haworth Press.

Chang S-S, Stuckler D, Yip P & Gunnel D (2013) Impact of 2008 global economic crisis on suicide: time trend in 54 countries. *British Medical Journal*, 347: f5239.

Chaplin R (2007) How can clinicians help patients to take their psychotropic medication? *Advances in Psychiatric Treatment*, 13(5): 347–349.

Chapman SCE & Horne R (2013) Medication nonadherence and psychiatry. *Current Opinion in Psychiatry*, 26(5): 446–452.

Charland LC (2006) Moral nature of the DSM-IV cluster B personality disorders. *Journal of Personality Disorders*, 20(2): 116–125.

Clark M (2015) Co-production in mental health care. *Mental Health Review Journal*, 20(4): 213–219.

Clements J & Davies E (2013) Prevention of psychosis: creating societies where more people flourish. In Read J & Dillon J (eds) *Models of Madness: Psychological, Social and Biological Approaches to Schizophrenia*, 2nd edition. Hove: Routledge, pp. 295–304.

Cohen D & Hughes S (2011) How do people taking psychiatric drugs explain their 'chemical imbalance?' *Ethical Human Psychology and Psychiatry*, 13(3): 176–189.

Cole S, Wood K & Spendelow J (2015) Team formulation: a critical evaluation of current literature and future research directions. *Clinical Psychology Forum*, 275: 13–19.

Coleman R (1999) *Recovery: An Alien Concept*. Gloucester: Handsell Publishing.

Coles S (2015) Meaning, madness and marginalisation. In Coles S, Keenan S & Diamond B (eds) *Madness Contested: Power and Practice*. Monmouth: PCCS Books, pp. 42–55.

Coles S, Keenan S & Diamond B (2015) Introduction. In Coles S, Keenan S & Diamond B (eds) *Madness Contested: Power and Practice*. Monmouth: PCCS Books, pp. vii–xvi.

Comer JS & Kendall PC (2013) Methodology, design, and evaluation in psychotherapy research. In Lambert MJ (ed) *Bergin and Garfield's Handbook of Psychotherapy and Behavior Change*, 6th edition. Hoboken, NJ: John Wiley & Sons, pp. 21–48.

Compton MT & Shim RS (eds) (2015) *The Social Determinants of Mental Health*. Arlington, VA: American Psychiatric Publishing.

Cooper M (2008) *Essential Research Findings in Counselling and Psychotherapy*. London: Sage.

Cooper M & McLeod J (2011) *Pluralistic Counselling and Psychotherapy*. London: Sage.

Copeland ME (1997) *Wellness Recovery Action Plan*. Dummerston, VT: Peach Press.

Correll CH, Detraux J, De Lepeleire J & De Hert M (2015) Effects of antipsychotics, antidepressants and mood stabilizers on risk for physical diseases in people with schizophrenia, depression and bipolar disorder. *World Psychiatry*, 14(2): 119–136.

Corrie S & Lane DA (2010) *Constructing Stories, Telling Tales: A Guide to Formulation in Applied Psychology*. London: Karnac Books.

Corstens D & Longden E (2013) The origins of voices: links between life history and voice hearing in a survey of 100 cases. *Psychosis*, 5(3): 270–285.

Corstens D, Longden E, McCarthy-Jones S ... Thomas N (2014) Emerging perspectives from the Hearing Voices Movement: implications for research and practice. *Schizophrenia Bulletin*, 40(suppl. 4): S285–S294.

Cottrell S (2017) *Critical Thinking Skills: Developing Effective Analysis and Argument*, 3rd edition. Basingstoke: Palgrave Macmillan.

Crawford MJ, Thana L, Farquharson L ... Parry GD (2016) Patient experience of negative effects of psychological treatment: results of a national survey. *The British Journal of Psychiatry*, 208(3): 260–265.

Crenshaw K (1989) Demarginalizing the intersection of race and sex: a black feminist critique of antidiscrimination doctrine, feminist theory and antiracist politics. *University of Chicago Legal Forum*, 1989(1): 139–167.

Cresswell M (2005) Psychiatric 'survivors' and testimonies of self-harm. *Social Science & Medicine*, 61(8): 1668–1677.

Crichton P, Carel H & Kidd IJ (2016) Epistemic injustice in psychiatry. *BJPsych Bulletin*, 41(3): 1–6.

Cromby J, Harper D & Reavey P (2013) Biology. In Cromby J, Harper D & Reavey P (eds) *Psychology, Mental Health and Distress*. Basingstoke: Palgrave Macmillan, pp. 75–100.

Crow TJ (2010) The continuum of psychosis – 1986–2010. *Psychiatric Annals*, 40(2): 115–119.

Cuijpers P, Berking M, Andersson G ... Dobson KS (2013) A meta-analysis of cognitive-behavioural therapy for adult depression, alone and in comparison with other treatments. *Canadian Journal of Psychiatry*, 58(7): 376–385.

Curtis T, Dellar R, Leslie E & Watson B (eds) (2000) *Mad Pride: A Celebration of Mad Culture*. London: Spare Change Books.

Darder A, Baltodano MP & Torres RD (eds) (2017) *The Critical Pedagogy Reader*, 3rd edition. New York, NY: Routledge.

Davidson L, Bellamy C, Guy K & Miller R (2012) Peer support among persons with severe mental illnesses: a review of evidence and experience. *World Psychiatry*, 11(2): 123–128.

Davidson L, Rakfeldt J & Strauss J (2010) *The Roots of the Recovery Movement in Psychiatry: Lessons Learned*. Chichester: John Wiley & Sons.

Deacon BJ (2013) The biomedical model of mental disorder: a critical analysis of its validity, utility, and effects on psychotherapy research. *Clinical Psychology Review*, 33(7): 846–861.

Deegan PE (1988) Recovery: the lived experience of rehabilitation. *Psychosocial Rehabilitation Journal*, 11(4): 11–19.

Deegan PE (1992) The independent living movement and people with psychiatric disabilities: taking back control over our own lives. *Psychosocial Rehabilitation Journal*, 15(3): 3–19.

Deegan PE (1993) Recovering our sense of value after being labeled mentally ill. *Journal of Psychosocial Nursing and Mental Health Services*, 31(4): 7–11.

Deegan PE (1996) Recovery as a journey of the heart. *Psychiatric Rehabilitation Journal*, 19(3): 91–97.

Deegan PE (2005) The importance of personal medicine: a qualitative study of resilience in people with psychiatric disabilities. *Scandinavian Journal of Public Health*, 33(66): 29–35.

Deegan PE & Drake RE (2006) Shared decision making and medication management in the recovery process. *Psychiatric Services*, 57(11): 1636–1639.

Deleuze G (2001/1968) *Difference and Repetition*. London: Continuum.

DeRosse P & Karlsgodt KH (2015) Examining the psychosis continuum. *Current Behavioral Nueroscience Reports*, 2(2): 80–89.

Dewey J (1980/1916) Democracy and education. In Boydston JA (ed) *John Dewey: The Middle Works, 1899–1924. Volume 9: 1916*. Carbondale, IL: Southern Illinois Press, pp. 1–370.

Dillon J (2010) The tale of an ordinary little girl. *Psychosis*, 2(1): 79–83.

Dillon J (2011) The personal is the political. In Rapley M, Moncrieff J & Dillon J (eds) *De-Medicalising Misery: Psychiatry, Psychology and the Human Condition*. Basingstoke: Palgrave Macmillan, pp. 141–157.

Dimidjian S & Hollon SD (2010) How would we know if psychotherapy were harmful? *American Psychologist*, 65(1): 21–33.

Diprose K (2015) Resilience is futile. *Soundings*, 58: 44–56.

Double D (2011) Why were doctors so slow to recognise antidepressant discontinuation problems. In Rapley M, Moncrieff J & Dillon J (eds) *De-Medicalising Misery: Psychiatry, Psychology and the Human Condition*. Basingstoke: Palgrave Macmillan, pp. 197–210.

Dragioti E, Dimoliatis I & Evangelou E (2015) Disclosure of researcher allegiance in meta-analyses and randomised controlled trials of psychotherapy: a systematic appraisal. *BMJ Open*, 5: e007206.

Duncan BL, Miller SD, Wampold BE & Hubble MA (2010) *The Heart and Soul of Change: Delivering What Works in Therapy*, 2nd edition. Washington, DC: American Psychological Association.

Ecclestone K & Hayes D (2009) *The Dangerous Rise of Therapeutic Education*. Abingdon: Routledge.

Edwards BM (2015) Recovery: accepting the unacceptable? *Clinical Psychology Forum*, 268: 16–27.

Ellahi R (2015) Serotonin syndrome: a spectrum of toxicity. *BJPsych Advances*, 21(5): 324–332.

Ellis A (1962) *Reason and Emotion in Psychotherapy*. New York, NY: Lyle Stuart.

Engel GL (1977) The need for a new medical model: a challenge for biomedicine. *Science*, 196(4286): 129–136.

Epictetus (2008) Enchiridion. In Dobbin R (ed) *Epictetus: Discourses and Selected Writings*. London: Penguin, pp. 219–245.

Epstein WM (1995) *The Illusion of Psychotherapy*. New Brunswick, NJ: Transaction Publishers.

Erhart SM, Marder SR & Carpenter WT (2006) Treatment of schizophrenia negative symptoms: future prospects. *Schizophrenia Bulletin*, 32(2): 234–237.

Even C, Sioubud-Dorocant E & Dardennes RM (2000) Critical approach to antidepressant trials: blindness protection is necessary, feasible and measurable. *British Journal of Psychiatry*, 177(1): 47–51.

Fairclough N (2015) *Language and Power*, 3rd edition. Abingdon: Routledge.

Faulkner A (2017) Survivor research and Mad Studies: the role and value of experiential knowledge in mental health research. *Disability & Society*, 32(4): 500–520.

Faulkner A & Kalathil J (2012) *The Freedom to Be, the Chance to Dream: Preserving User-led Peer Support in Mental Health*. London: Together for Mental Wellbeing.

Faulkner A, Yiannoullou S, Kalathil J ... Kallevik J (2015) *Involvement for Influence: The 4Pi Standards for Involvement*. London: NSUN.

Fernando S (2008) Institutional racism and cultural diversity. In Tummey R & Turner T (eds) *Critical Issues in Mental Health*. Basingstoke: Palgrave Macmillan, pp. 41–57.

Fernando S (2010) *Mental Health, Race and Culture*, 3rd edition. Basingstoke: Palgrave Macmillan.

Fernando S (2017) *Institutional Racism in Psychiatry and Clinical Psychology: Race Matters in Mental Health*. London. Palgrave Macmillan.

Ferraro D (2016) Psychology in the age of austerity. *Psychotherapy and Politics International*, 14(1): 17–24.

Fetridge MA, Milner R, Gavin V & Levita L (2015) Borderline personality disorder: patterns of self-harm, reported childhood trauma and clinical outcome. *British Journal of Psychiatry Open*, 1(1): 18–20.

Filson B (2016) The haunting can end: trauma-informed approaches in healing from abuse and adversity. In Russo J & Sweeney A (eds) *Searching for a Rose Garden: Challenging Psychiatry, Fostering Mad Studies*. Monmouth: PCCS Books, pp. 20–24.

Filson B & Mead S (2016) Becoming part of each other's narratives: Intentional Peer Support. In Russo J & Sweeney A (eds) *Searching for a Rose Garden: Challenging Psychiatry, Fostering Mad Studies*. Monmouth: PCCS Books, pp. 109–117.

Fisher A (2011) *Critical Thinking: An Introduction*, 2nd edition. Cambridge: Cambridge University Press.

Fisher HL, Craig TK, Fearon P ... Morgan C (2011) Reliability and comparability of psychosis patients' retrospective reports of childhood abuse. *Schizophrenia Bulletin*, 37(3): 546–553.

Fitzpatrick R, Kumar S, Nkansa-Dwamena O & Thorne L (2014) *Ethnic Inequalities in Mental Health: Promoting Lasting Positive Change*. London: Lankelly Chase Foundation.

Fosse R, Joseph J & Jones M (2016) Schizophrenia: a critical view on genetic effects. *Psychosis*, 8(1): 72–84.

Fosse R, Joseph J & Richardson K (2015) A critical assessment of the equal-environment assumption of the twin method for schizophrenia. *Frontiers in Psychiatry*, 6(62): 1–10.

Foucault M (1981) The order of discourse. In Young R (ed) *Untying the Text: A Post-Structuralist Reader*. Boston, MA: Routledge & Kegan Paul, pp. 51–78.

Foucault M (1990) Practising criticism. In Kritzman LD (ed) *Michel Foucault. Politics, Philosophy, Culture: Interviews and Other Writings 1977–1984*. New York: Routledge, pp. 152–156.

Foucault M (2001/1961) *Madness and Civilization: A History of Insanity in the Age of Reason*. London: Routledge.

Foucault M (2002) Questions of method. In Faubion JD (ed) *Power: Essential Works of Foucault: 1954–1984. Volume 3*. London: Penguin, pp. 223–238.

Foucault M (2005/1966) *The Order of Things: An Archaeology of the Human Sciences*. London: Routledge.

Frances A (2013) *Saving Normal: An Insider's Revolt Against Out-of-Control Psychiatric Diagnosis, DSM-5, Big Pharma, and the Medicalization of Ordinary Life*. New York, NY: William Morrow.

Freire P (1970) *Pedagogy of the Oppressed*. New York, NY: Herder & Herder.

Fricker M (2007) *Epistemic Injustice: Power and the Ethics and Knowing*. Oxford: Oxford University Press.

Fricker M (2008) FORUM: Miranda Fricker's epistemic injustice: power and the ethics of knowing. *THEORIA*: 23(1): 69–71.

Friedli L (2009) *Mental Health, Resilience and Inequalities*. Copenhagen: World Health Organization.

Fromm E (1955) *The Sane Society*. New York, NY: Rinehart & Company.

Frueh CB, Knapp RG, Cusak KJ ... Hiers TG (2005) Patients' reports of traumatic or harmful experiences within the psychiatric setting. *Psychiatric Services*, 56(9): 1123–1133.

Fulford KWM, Broome M, Stanghellini G & Thornton T (2005) Looking with both eyes open: fact *and* value in psychiatric diagnosis? *World Psychiatry*, 4(2): 78–86.

Furedi F (2004) *Therapy Culture: Cultivating Vulnerability in an Uncertain Age*. London: Routledge.

Fusar-Poli P, Smieskova R, Kempton MJ ... Borgwardt S (2013) Progressive brain changes in schizophrenia related to antipsychotic treatment? A meta-analysis of longitudinal MRI studies. *Neuroscience and Biobehavioral Reviews*, 37(8): 1680–1691.

Geller JL (2012) Patient-centered, recovery-orientated psychiatric care and treatment are not always voluntary. *Psychiatric Services*, 63(5): 493–495.

Gergen KJ (1990) Therapeutic professions and the diffusion of deficit. *Journal of Mind and Behavior*, 11(3–4): 353–368.

Gibson K, Cartwright C & Read J (2016) 'In my life antidepressants have been ...': a qualitative analysis of users' diverse experiences with antidepressants. *BMC Psychiatry*, 16(135): 1–7.

Goldsmith LP, Lewis SW, Dunn G & Bentall RP (2015) Psychological treatments for early psychosis can be beneficial or harmful, depending on the therapeutic alliance: an instrumental variable analysis. *Psychological Medicine*, 45(11): 2365–2373.

Gonzales L, Davidoff KC, Nadal KL & Yanos PT (2015) Microaggressions experienced by persons with mental illnesses: an exploratory study. *Psychiatric Rehabilitation Journal*, 38(3): 234–241.

Gosling J (2010) The ethos of involvement as the route to recovery. In Weinstein J (ed) *Mental Health, Service User Involvement and Recovery*. London: Jessica Kingsley Publishers, pp. 30–39.

Gøtzsche PC (2013) *Deadly Medicines and Organised Crime: How Big Pharma Has Corrupted Healthcare*. London: Radcliffe Publishing.

Gøtzsche PC, Young AH & Grace J (2015) Does long term use of psychiatric drugs cause more harm than good? *British Medical Journal*, 350: h2435.

Greenberg G (2013) *The Book of Woe: The DSM and the Unmaking of Psychiatry*. New York, NY: Blue Rider Press.

Greenhalgh T (2014) *How to Read a Paper: The Basics of Evidence-Based Medicine*, 5th edition. Chichester: John Wiley & Sons.

Gunn JS & Potter B (2015) *Borderline Personality Disorder: New Perspectives on a Stigmatizing and Overused Diagnosis*. Santa Barbara: Praeger.

Guyatt G, Rennie D, Meade MO & Cook DJ (eds) (2015) *Users' Guide to the Medical Literature: Essentials of Evidence-Based Clinical Practice*, 3rd edition. New York, NY: McGraw-Hill Education.

Habermas J (1972) *Knowledge and Human Interests*. Boston, MA: Beacon Press.

Hallett K (2015) Intersectionality and serious mental illness – a case study and recommendations for practice. *Women & Therapy*, 38(1–2): 156–174.

Hanscomb S (2017) *Critical Thinking: The Basics*. London: Routledge.

Hare W (2007) What is open-mindedness? In Hare W & Portelli JP (eds) *Key Questions for Educators*. San Francisco, CA: Caddo Gap Press, pp. 21–24.

Hare W (2011) Helping open-mindedness flourish. *Journal of Thought*, 46(1–2): 9–10.

Harper D & Speed E (2012) Uncovering recovery: the resistible rise of recovery and resilience. *Studies in Social Justice*, 6(1): 9–26.

Harris M & Fallot RD (2001) Envisioning a trauma-informed service system: a vital paradigm shift. *New Directions for Mental Health Services*, 89: 3–22.

Harrison E (2013) Bouncing back? Recession, resilience and everyday lives. *Critical Social Policy*, 33(1): 97–113.

Harrow M & Jobe TH (2013) Does long-term treatment of schizophrenia with antipsychotic medications facilitate recovery? *Schizophrenia Bulletin*, 39(5): 962–965.

Harvey D (2007) *A Brief History of Neoliberalism*. Oxford: Oxford University Press.

Haw C, Hawton K, Gunnell & Platt S (2016) Economic recession and suicidal behaviour: possible mechanisms and ameliorating factors. *International Journal of Social Psychiatry*, 61(1): 73–81.

Healey D (2014) The cardinals of psychiatry. In Speed E, Moncrieff J & Rapley M (eds) *De-Medicalising Misery II: Society, Politics and the Mental Health Industry*. Basingstoke: Palgrave Macmillan, pp. 174–189.

Healey D (2016) *Psychiatric Drugs Explained*, 6th edition. London: Elsevier.

Heath M (2012) On critical thinking. *The International Journal of Narrative Therapy and Community Work*, 4: 11–18.

Hempel CG (1994) Fundamentals of taxonomy. In Sadler JZ, Wiggins OP & Schwartz MA (eds) *Philosophical Perspectives on Psychiatric Classification*. Baltimore, MD: John Hopkins University Press, pp. 315–331.

Herman J (2015) *Trauma and Recovery: The Aftermath of Violence – From Domestic Abuse to Political Terror*. New York, NY: Basic Books.

Hirschfeld RMA (2000) History and evolution of the monoamine hypothesis of depression. *Journal of Clinical Psychiatry*, 61(suppl 6): 4–6.

Hitchen S, Watkins M, Williamson GR ... Taylor M (2011) Lone voices have an emotional content: focussing on mental health service user and carer involvement. *International Journal of Health Care Quality Assurance*, 24(2): 164–177.

Ho BC, Andreasen NC, Ziebell S ... Magnotta V (2011) Long-term antipsychotic treatment and brain volumes: a longitudinal study of first-episode schizophrenia. *Archives of General Psychiatry*, 68(2): 128–137.

Hoff P (2015) The Kraepelinian tradition. *Dialogues in Clinical Neuroscience*, 17(1): 31–41.

Hofmann SG, Asnaani A, Imke JJ ... Fang A (2012) The efficacy of cognitive behavioral therapy: a review of meta-analyses. *Cognitive Therapy and Research*, 36(5): 427–440.

Holland K (2018) *Cultural Awareness in Nursing and Health Care: An Introductory Text*, 3rd edition. New York, NY: Routledge.

Holmes G (2015) Toxic mental environments and other psychology in the real world groups. In Coles S, Keenan S & Diamond B (eds) *Madness Contested: Power and Practice*. Monmouth: PCCS Books, pp. 247–266.

Honos-Webb L & Leitner LM (2001) How using the DSM causes damage: a client's report. *Journal of Humanistic Psychology*, 41(4): 36–56.

Houghton JF (1982) Maintaining mental health in a turbulent world. *Schizophrenia Bulletin*, 8(3): 548–552.

Howell A & Veronka J (2012) Introduction: the politics of resilience and recovery in mental health care. *Studies in Social Justice*, 6(1): 1–7.

Howes OD & Kapur S (2009) The dopamine hypothesis of schizophrenia: version III – the final common pathway. *Schizophrenia Bulletin*, 35(3): 549–562.

Hunsley J & Di Giulio G (2002) Dodo bird, phoenix, or urban legend? The question of psychotherapy equivalence. *The Scientific Review of Mental Health Practice*, 1(1): 11–22.

Hyman SE & Nestler EJ (1996) Initiation and adaptation: a paradigm for understanding psychotropic drug action. *American Journal of Psychiatry*, 153(2): 151–162.

Inckle K (2017) *Safe with Self-Injury: A Practical Guide to Understanding, Responding and Harm Reduction.* Monmouth: PCCS Books.

Ingram RA (2016) Doing Mad Studies: making (non)sense together. *Intersectionalities*, 5(3): 11–17.

Insel TR (2009) Disruptive insights in psychiatry: transforming a clinical discipline. *The Journal of Clinical Investigation*, 119(4): 700–705.

Insel TR (2015) A different way of thinking. *New Scientist*, 227(3035): 5.

Insel TR & Cuthbert BN (2015) Brain disorders? Precisely. *Science*, 348(6234): 499–500.

Jackson V (2002) In our own voice: African-American stories of oppression, survival and recovery in mental health systems. *International Journal of Narrative Therapy and Community Work*, 2002(2): 11–31.

Johnsen TJ & Friborg O (2015) The effects of cognitive behavioral therapy as an anti-depressive treatment is falling: a meta-analysis. *Psychological Bulletin*, 141(4): 747–768.

Johnstone L (2000) *Users and Abusers of Psychiatry: A Critical Look at Psychiatric Practice*, 2nd edition. London: Routledge.

Johnstone L (2008) Psychiatric diagnosis. In Tummey R & Turner T (eds) *Critical Issues in Mental Health*. Basingstoke: Palgrave Macmillan, pp. 5–22.

Johnstone L (2012) Do families cause 'schizophrenia?' Revisiting a taboo subject. In Newnes C, Holmes G & Dunn C (eds) *This is Madness: A Critical Look at Psychiatry and the Future of Mental Health Services*. Ross-on-Wye: PCCS Books, pp. 119–134.

Johnstone L (2013) Diagnosis and formulation. In Cromby J, Harper D & Reavey P (eds) *Psychology, Mental Health and Distress*. Basingstoke: Palgrave Macmillan, pp. 101–117.

Johnstone L & Dallos R (eds) (2014) *Formulation in Psychology and Psychotherapy: Making Sense of People's Problems*, 2nd edition. Hove: Routledge.

Jones PB, Barnes TR, Davies L ... Lewis SW (2006) Randomized controlled trial of the effect on quality of life of second- vs. first-generation antipsychotic drugs in schizophrenia. Cost utility of the latest antipsychotic drugs in schizophrenia study (CUtLASS 1). *Archives of General Psychiatry*, 63(10): 1079–1087.

Joseph J (2013) 'Schizophrenia' and heredity: why the emperor (still) has no genes. In Read J & Dillon J (eds) *Models of Madness: Psychological, Social and Biological Approaches to Schizophrenia*, 2nd edition. Hove: Routledge, pp. 72–89.

Joseph J (2015) *The Trouble with Twin Studies: A Reassessment of Twin Research in the Social and Behavioral Sciences*. New York, NY: Routledge.

Kain KL & Terrell SJ (2018) *Nurturing Resilience: Helping Clients Move Forward from Developmental Trauma*. Berkeley, CA: North Atlantic Books.

Kaminskiy E, Ramon S & Morant N (2013) Exploring shared decision making for psychiatric medication management. In Walker S (ed) *Modern Mental Health: Critical Perspectives on Psychiatric Practice*. St Albans: Critical Publishing, pp. 33–48.

Kapur S, Agid O, Mizrahi R & Li M (2006) How antipsychotics work – from receptors to reality. *NeuroRx*, 3(1): 10–21.

Kendall T (2011) The rise and fall of the atypical antipsychotics. *British Journal of Psychiatry*, 199(4): 266–268.

Kendler KS (2005) Toward a philosophical structure for psychiatry. *American Journal of Psychiatry*, 162(3): 433–440.

Kendler KS (2008) Explanatory models for psychiatric illness. *American Journal of Psychiatry*, 165(6): 695–702.

Kendler KS (2014) The structure of psychiatric science. *American Journal of Psychiatry*, 171(9): 931–938.

Kennerley H, Kirk J & Westbrook D (2016) *An Introduction to Cognitive Behaviour Therapy: Skills and Applications*, 3rd edition. London: Sage.

Keshavan MS, Morris DW, Sweeney JA ... Tamminga C (2011) A dimensional approach to the psychosis spectrum between bipolar disorder and schizophrenia: the Schizo-Bipolar Scale. *Schizophrenia Research*, 133(1–3): 250–254.

Kessler RC, McLaughlin KA, Green JG ... Williams DR (2010) Childhood adversities and adult psychopathology in the WHO World Mental Health Surveys. *British Journal of Psychiatry*, 197(5): 378–385.

Kidd IJ & Carel H (2017) Epistemic injustice and illness. *Journal of Applied Philosophy*, 34(2): 172–190.

Kinderman P (2014) *A Prescription for Psychiatry: Why We Need a Whole New Approach to Mental Health and Wellbeing*. Basingstoke. Palgrave Macmillan.

King C (2016) Whiteness in psychiatry: the madness of European misdiagnoses. In Russo J & Sweeney A (eds) *Searching for a Rose Garden: Challenging Psychiatry, Fostering Mad Studies*. Monmouth: PCCS Books, pp. 69–76.

King G (2014) Staff attitudes towards people with borderline personality disorder. *Mental Health Practice*, 17(5): 30–34.

King LS (1954) What is disease? *Philosophy of Science*, 21(3): 193–203.

Kirkbride JB, Jones PB, Ullrich S & Coid JW (2014) Social deprivation, inequality, and the neighborhood-level incidence of psychotic syndromes in East London. *Schizophrenia Bulletin*, 40(1): 169–180.

Kirsch I (2011) Antidepressants and the placebo response. In Rapley M, Moncrieff J & Dillon J (eds) *De-Medicalising Misery: Psychiatry, Psychology and the Human Condition*. Basingstoke: Palgrave Macmillan, pp. 189–196.

Kirsch I (2014) Antidepressants and the placebo effect. *Zeitschrift für Psychologie*, 222(3): 128–134.

Klerman GL (1978) The evolution of a scientific nosology. In Shershow JC (ed) *Schizophrenia: Science and Practice*. Cambridge, MA: Harvard University Press, pp. 99–121.

Kloos B, Hill J, Thomas E ... Dalton JH (2012) *Community Psychology: Linking Individuals and Communities*, 3rd edition. Belmont, CA: Wadsworth, Cengage Learning.

Knowles SF, Hearne J & Smith I (2015) Physical restraint and the therapeutic relationship. *The Journal of Forensic Psychiatry and Psychology*, 26(4): 461–475.

Kornhuber J, Riederer P, Reynolds GP ... Gabriel E (1989) 3H-spiperone binding sites in post-mortem brains from schizophrenic patients: relationship to neuroleptic drug treatment, abnormal movements and positive symptoms. *Journal of Neural Transmission*, 75(1): 1–10.

Lacasse JR & Leo J (2005) Serotonin and depression: a disconnect between the advertisements and the scientific literature. *PLoS Medicine*, 2(12): e392.

Lacasse JR & Leo J (2015) Antidepressants and the chemical imbalance theory of depression: a reflection and update on the discourse. *the Behavior Therapist*, 38(7): 206–213.

Laing RD (1960) *The Divided Self*. London: Tavistock Publications.

Laing RD (1967) *The Politics of Experience and The Bird of Paradise*. London: Penguin.

Lake RC (2012) *Schizophrenia is a Misdiagnosis: Implications for the DSM-5 and the ICD-11*. New York: Springer.

Lakeman R (2014) The Finnish open dialogue approach to crisis intervention in psychosis: a review. *Psychotherapy in Australia*, 20(3): 26–33.

Lambert MJ (2013) The efficacy and effectiveness of psychotherapy. In Lambert MJ (ed) *Bergin and Garfield's Handbook of Psychotherapy and Behavior Change*, 6th edition. Hoboken, NJ: John Wiley & Sons, pp. 169–218.

Leamy M, Bird V, Le Boutillier C ... Slade M (2011) Conceptual framework for personal recovery in mental health: systematic review and narrative synthesis. *The British Journal of Psychiatry*, 199(6): 445–452.

Lee T & Seeman P (1980) Elevation of brain/neuroleptic receptors in schizophrenia. *American Journal of Psychiatry*, 137(2): 191–197.

Leete E (1989) How I perceive and mange my illness. *Schizophrenia Bulletin*, 15(2): 197–200.

LeFrançois BA, Menzies R & Reaume G (eds) (2013) *Mad Matters: A Critical Reader in Canadian Mad Studies*. Toronto: Canadian Scholars' Press.

Leising D, Rogers K & Ostner J (2009) The undisordered personality: normative assumptions underlying personality disorder diagnoses. *Review of General Psychology*, 13(3): 230–241.

Leucht S, Cipriani A, Spineli L ... Davis JM (2013) Comparative efficacy and tolerability of 15 antipsychotic drugs in schizophrenia: a multiple-treatments meta-analysis. *The Lancet*, 382(9896): 951–962.

Lewis S & Lieberman J (2008) CATIE and CUtLASS: can we handle the truth? *The British Journal of Psychiatry*, 192(3): 161–163.

Lieberman JA (2016) *Shrinks: The Untold Story of Psychiatry*. London: Weidenfeld & Nicolson.

Lilienfeld SO (2007) Psychological treatments that cause harm. *Perspectives on Psychological Science*, 2(1): 53–70.

Linden M & Schermuly-Haupt ML (2014) Definition, assessment and rate of psychotherapy side effects. *World Psychiatry*, 13(3): 306–309.

Lindow V (2012) Survivor-controlled alternatives to psychiatric services. In Newnes C, Holmes G & Dunn C (eds) *This is Madness: A Critical Look at Psychiatry and the Future of Mental Health Services*. Ross-on-Wye: PCCS Books, pp. 211–226.

Linscott RJ & van Os J (2013) An updated and conservative systematic review and meta-analysis of epidemiological evidence on psychotic experiences in children and adults: on the pathway from proneness to persistence to dimensional expression factors across mental disorders. *Psychological Medicine*, 43(6): 1133–1149.

Lloyd-Evans B, Mayo-Wilson E, Harrison B ... Kendall T (2014) A systematic review and meta-analysis of randomised controlled trials of peer support for people with severe mental illness. *BMC Psychiatry*, 14(39): 1–12.

Longden E (2010) Making sense of voices: a personal story of recovery. *Psychosis*, 2(3): 255–259.

Longden E, Corstens D, Escher S & Romme M (2012) Voice hearing in biographical context: a model for formulating the relationship between voices and life history. *Psychosis*, 4(3): 224–234.

Looi GME, Engström Å & Sävenstedt S (2015) A self-destructive care: self-report of people who experienced coercive measures and their suggestions for alternatives. *Issues in Mental Health Nursing*, 36(2): 96–103.

Luborsky L, Rosenthal R, Diguer L ... Krause ED (2002) The dodo bird verdict is alive and well – mostly. *Clinical Psychology: Science and Practice*, 9(1): 2–12.

Luborsky L, Singer B & Luborsky L (1975) Comparative studies of psychotherapies: is it true that 'Everyone has won and all must have prizes'? *Archive of General Psychiatry*, 32(8): 995–1008.

Luciano M, Sampogna G, Del Vecchio V ... Fiorillo A (2014) Use of coercive measures in mental health practice and its impact on outcome: a critical review. *Expert Review of Neurotherapeutics*, 14(2): 131–141.

Lynch T (2015) *Depression Delusion, Volume One: The Myth of the Brain Chemical Imbalance*. Limerick: Mental Health Publishing.

Mackay AVP, Iverson LL, Rossor M ... Snyder SH (1982) Increased brain dopamine and dopamine receptors in schizophrenia. *Archives of General Psychiatry*, 39(9): 991–997.

Malla A, Joober R & Garcia A (2015) 'Mental illness is like any other medical illness': a critical examination of the statement and its impact on patient care and society. *Journal of Psychiatry and Neuroscience*, 40(3): 147–150.

Marcus DK, O'Connell D, Norris AL & Sawaqdeh A (2014) Is the Dodo bird endangered in the 21st century? A meta-analysis of treatment comparison studies. *Clinical Psychology Review*, 34(7): 519–530.

Masson J (1988) *Against Therapy: Emotional Tyranny and the Myth of Psychological Healing*. New York: Atheneum.

Matthias MS, Salyers MP, Rollins AL & Frankel RM (2012) Decision making in recovery-oriented mental health care. *Psychiatric Rehabilitation Journal*, 35(4): 305–314.

May R (1950) *The Meaning of Anxiety*. New York, NY: The Ronald Press Company.

May R, Smith R, Ashton S ... Bull P (2015) Speaking out against the apartheid approach to our minds. In Coles S, Keenan S & Diamond B (eds) *Madness Contested: Power and Practice*. Monmouth: PCCS Books, pp. 233–246.

McHugh RK, Whitton SW, Peckham AD, ... Otto MW (2013) Patient preference for psychological vs. pharmacological treatment of psychiatric disorders: a meta-analytic review. *Journal of Clinical Psychiatry*, 74(6): 595–602.

McKeith J & Burns S (2011) *The Recovery Star: User Guide*, 2nd edition. London: Mental Health Providers Forum.

McLaughlin P, Giacco D & Priebe (2016) Use of coercive measures during involuntary psychiatric admission and treatment outcomes: data from a prospective study across 10 European countries. *PLoS ONE*, 11(12): e0168720.

McWade B (2016) Recovery-as-policy as a form of neoliberal state making. *Intersectionalities*, 5(3): 62–81.

Menzies R, LeFrançois BA & Reaume G (2013) Introducing Mad Studies. In LeFrançois BA, Menzies R & Reaume G (eds) *Mad Matters: A Critical Reader in Canadian Mad Studies*. Toronto: Canadian Scholars' Press Inc, pp. 1–22.

Mezirow J (1997) Transformative learning: theory to practice. *New Directions for Adult and Continuing Education*, 74: 5–12.

Miller DD, Caroff SN, Davis SM ... Lieberman JA (2008) Extrapyramidal side-effects of antipsychotics in a randomised trial. *The British Journal of Psychiatry*, 193(4): 279–288.

Mills C (2014) *Decolonizing Global Mental Health: The Psychiatrization of the Majority World*. Hove: Routledge.

Mitchell AJ & Selmes T (2007) Why don't patients take their medicine? Reasons and solutions in psychiatry. *Advances in Psychiatric Treatment*, 13(5): 336–346.

Mizock L & Russinova Z (2015) Intersectional stigma and the acceptance process of women with mental illness. *Women & Therapy*, 38(1–2): 14–30.

Mizrahi R, Bagby RM, Zipursky RB & Kapur S (2005) How antipsychotics work: the patients' perspective. *Progress in Neuropsychopharmacology and Biological Psychiatry*, 29(5): 859–864.

Mohtashemi R, Stevens J, Jackson PG & Weatherhead S (2016) Psychiatrists' understanding and use of psychological formulation: a qualitative exploration. *BJPsych Bulletin*, 40(4): 212–216.

Moloney P (2013) *The Therapy Industry: The Irresistible Rise of the Talking Cure, and Why It Doesn't Work*. London: Pluto Press.

Moncrieff J (2008) *The Myth of the Chemical Cure: A Critique of Psychiatric Drug Treatment*. Basingstoke: Palgrave Macmillan.

Moncrieff J (2009) *A Straight Talking Introduction to Psychiatric Drugs*. Ross-on-Wye: PCCS Books.

Moncrieff J (2010) Psychiatric diagnosis as a political device. *Social Theory & Health*, 8(4): 370–382.

Moncrieff J (2013) Psychiatric medication. In Cromby J, Harper D & Reavey P (eds) *Psychology, Mental Health and Distress*. Basingstoke: Palgrave Macmillan, pp. 160–168.

Moncrieff J (2015) The myths and realities of drug treatment for mental disorders. *the Behavior Therapist*, 38(7): 214–218.

Moncrieff J & Cohen D (2009) How do psychiatric drugs work? *British Medical Journal*, 338: 1535–1537.

Moncrieff J, Cohen D & Mason J (2015) The patient's dilemma: an analysis of users' experiences of taking neuroleptic drugs. In Coles S, Keenan S & Diamond B (eds) *Madness Contested: Power and Practice*. London: Hodder Arnold, pp. 213–232.

Moore TJ & Furberg CD (2016) The harms of antipsychotic drugs: evidence from key studies. *Drug Safety*, (40)1: 3–14.

Moos RH (2005) Iatrogenic effects of psychosocial interventions for substance use disorders: prevalence, predictors, prevention. *Addiction*, 100(5): 595–604.

Morant N, Kaminskiy E & Ramon S (2016) Shared decision making for psychiatric medication management: beyond the micro-social. *Health Expectations*, 19(5): 1002–1014.

Morgan A & Felton A (2015) From constructive engagement to coerced recovery. In Coles S, Keenan S & Diamond B (eds) *Madness Contested: Power and Practice*. Monmouth: PCCS Books, pp. 56–73.

Morgan G (2006) *Images of Organization*, 4th edition. Thousand Oaks, CA: Sage.

Morgan S (2013) *Risk Decision-Making: Working with Risk and Implementing Positive Risk-Taking*. Hove: Pavilion.

Moritsugu J, Vera E, Wong FY & Duffy KG (2016) *Community Psychology*, 5th edition. New York, NY: Routledge.

Morrow M (2013) Recovery: progressive paradigm or neoliberal smokescreen. In LeFrançois BA, Menzies R & Reaume G (eds) *Mad Matters: A Critical Reader in Canadian Mad Studies*. Toronto: Canadian Scholars' Press Inc, pp. 323–333.

Mosher LR, Hendrix V & Fort DC (2004) *Soteria: Through Madness to Deliverance*. San Francisco, CA: XLibris.

Mosher LR, Vallone R & Menn A (1995) The treatment of acute psychosis without neuroleptics: six-week psychopathology outcome data from the Soteria project. *International Journal of Social Psychiatry*, 41(3): 157–173.

Mulinari S (2012) Monoamine theories of depression: historical impact on biomedical research. *Journal of the History of the Neurosciences*, 21(4): 366–392.

Munder T, Brütsch O, Leonhart R … Barth J (2013) Researcher allegiance in psychotherapy outcome research: an overview of reviews. *Clinical Psychology Review*, 33(4): 501–511.

Nelson G & Prilleltensky I (eds) (2010) *Community Psychology: In Pursuit of Liberation and Well-being*, 2nd edition. Basingstoke: Palgrave Macmillan.

Nestler EJ, Pena CJ, Kundakovic M … Akbarian S (2016) Epigenetic basis of mental illness. *The Neuroscientist*, 22(2): 447–463.

Newnes C (2014) The Diagnostic and Statistical Manual: a history of critiques of psychiatric classification systems. In Speed E, Moncrieff J & Rapley M (eds) *De-Medicalising Misery II: Society, Politics and the Mental Health Industry*. Basingstoke: Palgrave Macmillan, pp. 190–209.

Norcross JC (ed) (2011) *Psychotherapy Relationships That Work: Evidence-Based Responsiveness*, 2nd edition. New York, NY: Oxford University Press.

Norcross JC & Lambert MJ (2011) Evidence-based therapy relationships. In Norcross JC (ed) *Psychotherapy Relationships That Work: Evidence-Based Responsiveness*, 2nd edition. New York, NY: Oxford University Press, pp. 3–21.

NSUN (National Service User Network) (2015) *The Language of Mental Wellbeing*. London: NSUN.

Nutt DJ & Sharpe M (2008) Uncritical positive regard? Issues in the efficacy and safety of psychotherapy. *Journal of Psychopharmacology*, 22(1): 3–6.

Ogles BM (2013) Measuring change in psychotherapy research. In Lambert MJ (ed) *Bergin and Garfield's Handbook of Psychotherapy and Behavior Change*, 6th edition. New Jersey: John Wiley & Sons, pp. 134–166.

O'Hagan M (2007) Parting thoughts. *Mental Notes*, 18: 4–5.

O'Hagan M (2014) *Madness Made Me: A Memoir*. Wellington: Open Box.

O'Hagan M (2016) Responses to a legacy of harm. In Russo J & Sweeney A (eds) *Searching for a Rose Garden: Challenging Psychiatry, Fostering Mad Studies*. Monmouth: PCCS Books, pp. 9–13.

Oliver M (2013) The social model of disability: thirty years on. *Disability & Society*, 28(7): 1024–1026.

Orford J (2008) *Community Psychology: Challenges, Controversies, and Emerging Consensus*. Chichester: John Wiley & Sons.

Palmier-Claus JE, Berry K, Bucci S … Varese F (2016) Relationship between childhood adversity and bipolar affective disorder: systematic review and meta-analysis. *The British Journal of Psychiatry*, 209(6): 454–459.

Parker C (2013) Antipsychotics in the treatment of schizophrenia. *Progress in Neurology and Psychiatry*, 17(3): 6–18.

Parry GD, Crawford MD & Duggan C (2016) Iatrogenic harm from psychological therapies – time to move on. *The British Journal of Psychiatry*, 208(3): 210–212.

Patel V, Collins PY, Copeland J … Skeen S (2011) The movement for global mental health. *British Journal of Psychiatry*, 198(2): 88–90.

Paul R & Elder L (2014) *Critical Thinking: Tools for Taking Charge of Your Professional and Personal Life*, 2nd edition. New Jersey: Pearson Education.

Pearlson GD (2015) Etiologic, phenomenologic, and endophenotypic overlap of schizophrenia and bipolar disorder. *Annual Review of Clinical Psychology*, 11: 251–281.

Pembroke LR (ed) (1995) *Self-Harm: Perspectives from Personal Experience*. London: Survivors Speak Out.

Penny D & Prescott L (2016) The co-optation of survivor knowledge: the danger of substituted values and voice. In Russo J & Sweeney A (eds) *Searching for a Rose Garden: Challenging Psychiatry, Fostering Mad Studies*. Monmouth: PCCS Books, pp. 35–45.

Perkins R (2015) Recovery: a journey of the mind and spirit. *Clinical Psychology Forum*, 268: 38–43.

Perkins R & Repper J (2013) Prejudice, discrimination and social exclusion: reducing the barriers to recovery for people diagnosed with mental health problems in the UK. *Neuropsychiatry*, 3(4): 377–384.

Peters ER, Williams SL, Cooke MA & Kuipers E (2012) It's not what you hear, it's the way you think about it: appraisals as determinants of affect and behaviour in voice hearers. *Psychological Medicine*, 42(7): 1507–1514.

Piaget J (1959) *The Language and Thought of the Child*. London: Routledge & Kegan Paul.

Pilgrim D (2014) The failure of modern psychiatry and some prospects of scientific progress offered by critical realism. In Speed E, Moncrieff J & Rapley M (eds) *De-Medicalising Misery II: Society, Politics and the Mental Health Industry*. Basingstoke: Palgrave Macmillan, pp. 58–75.

Pilgrim D & McCranie A (2013) *Recovery and Mental Health: A Critical Sociological Account*. Basingstoke: Palgrave Macmillan.

Pilgrim D & Rogers A (2008) Socioeconomic disadvantage. In Tummey R & Turner T (eds) *Critical Issues in Mental Health*. Basingstoke: Palgrave Macmillan, pp. 23–40.

Pitt L, Kilbride M, Welford M … Morrison AP (2009) Impact of a diagnosis of psychosis: user-led qualitative study. *BJPsych Bulletin*, 33(11): 419–423.

Plato, *Phaedrus*, in Hamiliton E & Cairns H (eds) *Plato: The Collected Dialogues*. Princeton, NJ: Princeton University Press, pp. 475–525.

Pramyothin P & Khaodhiar L (2010) Metabolic syndrome with the atypical antipsychotics. *Current Opinion in Endocrinology, Diabetes and Obesity*, 17(5): 460–466.

Prilleltensky I (1994) *The Morals and Politics of Psychology: Psychological Discourse and the Status Quo*. Albany, NY: State University of New York Press.

Proctor G (2007) Disordered boundaries? A critique of 'borderline personality disorder'. In Spandler H & Warner S (eds) *Beyond Fear and Control: Working with Young People who Self-Harm*. Ross-on-Wye: PCCS Books, pp. 105–118.

Proctor G (2017) *The Dynamics of Power in Counselling and Psychotherapy: Ethics, Politics and Practice*, 2nd edition. Monmouth: PCCS Books.

Rabkin JG, Markowitz JS, Stewart J … Klein DF (1986) How blind is blind? Assessment of patient and doctor medication guesses in a placebo-controlled trial of imipramine and phenelzine. *Psychiatry Research*, 19(1): 75–86.

Rapp CA & Goscha RJ (2012) *The Strengths Model: A Recovery-Orientated Approach to Mental Health Services*, 3rd edition. New York, NY: Oxford University Press.

Rappaport J (1977) *Community Psychology: Values, Research, and Action*. New York, NY: Holt, Rinehart and Winston.

Read J (2005) The bio-bio-bio model of madness. *The Psychologist*, 18(10): 596–597.

Read J (2009) *Psychiatric Drugs: Key Issues and Service User Perspectives*. Basingstoke: Palgrave Macmillan.

Read J & Bentall RP (2012) Negative childhood experiences and mental health: theoretical, clinical and primary prevention implications. *The British Journal of Psychiatry*, 200(2): 89–91.

Read J & Bentall RP (2013) Madness. In Cromby J, Harper D & Reavey P (eds) *Psychology, Mental Health and Distress*. Basingstoke: Palgrave Macmillan, pp. 249–282.

Read J, Fink PJ, Rudegeair T … Whitfield CL (2008) Child maltreatment and psychosis: a return to a genuinely integrated bio-psycho-social model. *Clinical Schizophrenia & Related Psychosis*, 2(3): 235–254.

Read J, Fosse R, Moskowitz A & Perry B (2014) The traumagenic neurodevelopmental model of psychosis revisited. *Neuropsychiatry*, 4(1): 65–79.

Read J, Hammersley P & Rudegeair T (2007) Why, when and how to ask about childhood abuse. *Advances in Psychiatric Treatment*, 13(2): 101–110.

Read J, Haslam N & Magliano L (2013) Prejudice, stigma and 'schizophrenia': the role of bio-genetic ideology. In Read J & Dillon J (eds) *Models of Madness: Psychological, Social and Biological Approaches to Psychosis*, 2nd edition. Hove: Routledge, pp. 157–177.

Read J, Haslam N, Sayce L & Davies E (2006) Prejudice and schizophrenia: a review of the 'mental illness is an illness like any other' approach. *Acta Psychiatrica Scandinavica*, 114(5): 303–318.

Read J & Reynolds J (eds) (1996) *Speaking Our Minds: An Anthology of Personal Experiences of Mental Distress and Its Consequences*. Basingstoke. Palgrave.

Read J & Sanders P (2011) *A Straight Talking Introduction to the Causes of Mental Health Problems*. Ross-on-Wye: PCCS Books.

Reber R (2016) *Critical Feeling: How to Use Feelings Strategically*. Cambridge: Cambridge University Press.

Reich SM, Riemer M, Prilleltensky I & Montero M (eds) (2007) *International Community Psychology: History and Theories*. New York, NY: Springer.

Reiff M, Castille DM, Muenzenmaier K & Link B (2012) Childhood abuse and the content of adult psychotic symptoms. *Psychological Trauma: Theory, Research, Practice, and Policy*, 4(4): 356–369.

Repper J & Carter T (2011) A review of the literature on peer support in mental health services. *Journal of Mental Health*, 20(4): 392–411.

Repper J & Perkins R (2012) Recovery: a journey of discovery for individuals and services. In Phillips P, Sandford T & Johnstone C (eds) *Working in Mental Health: Practice and Policy in a Changing Environment*. Abingdon: Routledge, pp. 71–80.

Richardson FC & Zeddies TJ (2001) Individualism and modern psychotherapy. In Slife BD, Williams RN & Barlow SH (eds) *Critical Issues in Psychotherapy: Translating New Ideas into Practice*. Thousand Oaks, CA: Sage, pp. 147–164.

Riordan HJ, Antonini P & Murphy MF (2011) Atypical antipsychotics and metabolic syndrome in patients with schizophrenia: risk factors, monitoring, and healthcare implications. *American Health & Drug Benefits*, 4(5): 292–302.

Roberts G & Boardman J (2013) Understanding 'recovery'. *Advances in Psychiatric Treatment*, 19(6): 400–409.

Roberts M (2008) Facilitating recovery by making sense of suffering: a Nietzschean perspective. *Journal of Psychiatric and Mental Health Nursing*, 15(9): 743–748.

Roberts M (2015) *Critical Thinking and Reflection for Mental Health Nursing Students*. London: Sage.

Roberts M & Ion R (2015) Thinking critically about the occurrence of widespread participation in poor nursing care. *Journal of Advanced Nursing*, 71(4): 768–776.

Rogers A & Pilgrim D (2014) *A Sociology of Mental Health and Illness*, 5th edition. Maidenhead: Open University Press.

Roiz-Santianez R, Suarez-Pinilla P & Crespo-Facorro B (2015) Brain structural effects of antipsychotic treatment in schizophrenia: a systematic review. *Current Neuropharmacology*, 13(4): 422–434.

Romme MA & Escher AD (1989) Hearing voices. *Schizophrenia Bulletin*, 15(2): 209–216.

Romme M & Escher S (eds) (1993) *Accepting Voices*. London: Mind Publications.

Romme M & Escher S (2000) *Making Sense of Voices: A Guide for Mental Health Professionals Working with Voice-Hearers*. London: Mind Publications.

Rose D (2001) *Users' Voices: The Perspectives of Mental Health Service Users on Community and Hospital Care*. London: Sainsbury Centre for Mental Health.

Rose D (2014) The mainstreaming of recovery. *Journal of Mental Health*, 23(5): 217–218.

Rose N (2003) Neurochemical selves. *Society*, 41(1): 46–59.

Rose S (2006) *The 21st-Century Brain: Explaining, Mending and Manipulating the Mind*. London: Vintage.

Rosenhan DL (1973) On being sane in insane places. *Science*, 179(4070): 250–258.

Rosenzweig S (1936) Some implicit common factors in diverse methods of psychotherapy: 'At last the Dodo said, "Everybody has won and all must have prizes"'. *American Journal of Orthopsychiatry*, 6(3): 412–415.

Rössler W, Ajdacic-Gross V, Müller M ... Hengartner MP (2015) Assessing sub-clinical psychosis phenotypes in the general population – a multidimensional approach. *Schizophrenia Research*, 161(2–3): 194–201.

Russo J (2016) Towards our own framework, or reclaiming madness part two. In Russo J & Sweeney A (eds) *Searching for a Rose Garden: Challenging Psychiatry, Fostering Mad Studies*. Monmouth: PCCS Books, pp. 59–68.

Russo J & Sweeney A (eds) (2016) *Searching for a Rose Garden: Challenging Psychiatry, Fostering Mad Studies*. Monmouth: PCCS Books.

Ryan W (1971) *Blaming the Victim*. New York, NY: Pantheon Books.

Sayce L (2016) *From Psychiatric Patient to Citizen Revisited*. London: Palgrave.

Scarr E, Millan MJ, Bahn S ... Dean B (2015) Biomarkers for psychiatry: the journey from fantasy to fact, a report of the 2013 CINP Think Tank. *International Journal of Neuropsychopharmacology*, 18(10): pyv042.

Schiraldi GR (2017) *The Resilience Workbook: Essential Skills to Recover from Stress, Trauma, and Adversity*. Oakland, CA: New Harbinger Publications.

Schomerus G, Schwahn C, Holzinger A ... Angermeyer MC (2012) Evolution of public attitudes about mental illness: a systematic review and meta-analysis. *Acta Psychiatrica Scandinavica*, 125(6): 440–452.

Schön DA (1983) *The Reflective Practitioner: How Professionals Think in Action*. New York, NY: Basic Books.

Schore AN (2001) The effects of early relational trauma on right brain development, affect regulation, and infant mental health. *Infant Mental Health Journal*, 22(1–2): 201–269.

Schore AN (2005) Attachment, affect regulation, and the developing right brain: linking developmental neuroscience to pediatrics. *Pediatrics in Review*, 26(6): 204–217.

Schore JR & Schore AN (2008) Modern attachment theory: the central role of affect regulation in development and treatment. *Clinical Social Work Journal*, 36(1): 9–20.

Scott J & Young AH (2016) Psychotherapies should be assessed for both benefit and harm. *The British Journal of Psychiatry*, 208(3): 208–209.

Scrutton AP (2017) Epistemic injustice and mental illness. In Kidd IJ, Medina J & Pohlhaus Jr., G (eds) *The Routledge Handbook of Epistemic Injustice*. Abingdon: Oxon, pp. 347–355.

Scull A (2011) *Hysteria: The Disturbing History*. Oxford: Oxford University Press.

Scull A (2016) *Madness in Civilization: A Cultural History of Insanity from the Bible to Freud, from the Madhouse to Modern Medicine*. London: Thames & Hudson.

Seale C, Chaplin R, Lelliott P & Quirk A (2006) Sharing decisions in consultations involving anti-psychotic medication: a qualitative study of psychiatrists' experiences. *Social Science & Medicine*, 62(11): 2861–2873.

Seale C, Chaplin R, Lelliott P & Quirk A (2007) Antipsychotic medication, sedation and mental clouding: an observational study of psychiatric consultations. *Social Science & Medicine*, 65(4): 698–711.

Sedgwick P (1982) *Psycho Politics*. London: Pluto Press.

Seikkula J (2015) Open dialogues with clients with mental health problems and their families. *Context*, 138: 2–6.

Shah J, Mizrahi R & McKenzie K (2011) The four dimensions: a model for the aetiology of psychosis. *The British Journal of Psychiatry*, 199(1): 11–14.

Shaw B (2015) Peer support. In Coles S, Keenan S & Diamond B (eds) *Madness Contested: Power and Practice*. Monmouth: PCCS Books, pp. 293–306.

Shaw C (2016) Deciding to be alive: self-injury and survival. In Russo J & Sweeney A (eds) *Searching for a Rose Garden: Challenging Psychiatry, Fostering Mad Studies*. Monmouth: PCCS Books, pp. 77–85.

Shim R, Koplan C, Langheim FJP ... Compton MT (2014) The social determinants of mental health: an overview and call to action. *Psychiatric Annals*, 44(1): 22–26.

Shorter E (1997) *A History of Psychiatry: From the Era of the Asylum to the Age of Prozac*. New York, NY: John Wiley & Sons.

SHRC (Scottish Human Rights Commission) (2016) *A Human Rights Based Approach to the Mental Health Strategy*. Edinburgh: SHRC.

Sibitz I, Scheutz A, Lakeman R ... Amering M (2011) Impact of coercive measures on life stories: qualitative study. *The British Journal of Psychiatry*, 199(3): 239–244.

Simpson A, Hannigan B, Coffey M ... Cartwright M (2016) Recovery-focused care planning and coordination in England and Wales: a cross-national mixed method comparative case study. *BMC Psychiatry*, 16(147): 1–18.

Sisti D, Young M & Caplan A (2013) Defining mental illnesses: can values and objectivity get along? *BMC Psychiatry*, 13: 346: 1–4.

Slade M (2009) *Personal Recovery and Mental Illness: A Guide for Mental Health Professionals*. Cambridge: Cambridge University Press.

Slade M, Amering M, Farkas M ...Whitley R (2014) Uses and abuses of recovery: implementing recovery-orientated practices in mental health systems. *World Psychiatry*, 13(1): 12–20.

Slade M & Wallace G (2017) Recovery and mental health. In Slade M, Oades L & Jarden A (eds) *Wellbeing, Recovery and Mental Health*. Cambridge: Cambridge University Press, pp. 24–34.

Slay J & Stephens L (2013) *Co-Production in Mental Health: A Literature Review*. London: New Economics Foundation.

Smail D (2011) Psychotherapy: illusion with no future? In Rapley M, Moncrieff J & Dillon J (eds) *De-Medicalising Misery: Psychiatry, Psychology and the Human Condition*. Basingstoke: Palgrave Macmillan, pp. 226–238.

Smail D (2014) *Power, Interest and Psychology: Elements of a Social Materialist Understanding of Distress*. Ross-on-Wye: PCCS Books.

Smail D (2015) *The Origins of Unhappiness: A New Understanding of Personal Distress*. London: Karnac Books.

Smith ML & Glass GV (1977) Meta-analysis of psychotherapy outcome studies. *American Psychologist*, 32(9): 752–760.

Southwick SM, Bonanno GA, Masten AS ... Yehuda R (2014) Resilience definitions, theory, and challenges: interdisciplinary perspectives. *European Journal of Psychotraumatology*, 5: 1–14.

Southwick SM & Charney DS (2012) *Resilience: The Science of Mastering Life's Greatest Challenges*. New York, NY: Cambridge University Press.

Spiegel JS (2012) Open-mindedness and intellectual humility. *Theory and Research in Education*, 10(1): 27–38.

Springer S (2016) *The Discourse of Neoliberalism: An Anatomy of a Powerful Idea*. London: Rowman & Littlefield.

Staddon P (ed) (2015) *Mental Health Service Users in Research: Critical Sociological Perspectives*. Bristol: Policy Press.

Stier M (2013) Normative preconditions for the assessment of mental disorder. *Frontiers in Psychology*, 4(611): 1–9.

Stiles WB, Barkham M, Mellor-Clark J & Connell J (2008) Effectiveness of cognitive-behavioural, person-centred, and psychodynamic therapies in UK primary-care routine practice: replication in a larger sample. *Psychological Medicine*, 38(5): 677–688.

Summerfield D (2012) Afterword: against 'global mental health'. *Transcultural Psychiatry*, 49(3): 519–530.

Sutton J (2007) *Healing the Hurt Within: Understand Self-Injury and Self-Harm, and Heal the Emotional Wounds*, 3rd edition. Oxford: How To Books Ltd.

Swatridge C (2014) *Oxford Guide to Effective Argument and Critical Thinking*. Oxford: Oxford University Press.

Sweeney A (2016) Why Mad Studies needs survivor research and why survivor research needs Mad Studies. *Intersectionalities*, 5(3): 36–61.

Sweeney A, Beresford P, Faulkner A ... Rose D (eds) (2009) *This is Survivor Research*. Ross-on-Wye: PCCS Books.

Sweeney A, Clement S, Filson B & Kennedy A (2016) Trauma-informed mental healthcare in the UK: what is it and how can we further its development? *Mental Health Review Journal*, 21(3): 174–192.

Sweeney A, Gillard S, Wykes T & Rose D (2015) The role of fear in mental health service users' experiences: a qualitative exploration. *Social Psychiatry and Psychiatric Epidemiology*, 50(7): 1079–1087.

Szasz TS (1960) The myth of mental illness. *American Psychologist*, 15(2): 113–118.

Szasz TS (1983) The myth of mental illness. In *Ideology and Insanity: Essays on the Psychiatric Dehumanization of Man*. London: Marion Boyars, pp. 12–24.

Thompson S & Thompson N (2008) *The Critically Reflective Practitioner*. Basingstoke: Palgrave Macmillan.

Thornicroft G (2006) *Shunned: Discrimination Against People with Mental Illness*. Oxford: Oxford University Press.

Thornton T (2007) *Essential Philosophy of Psychiatry*. Oxford: Oxford University Press.

Timimi S (2014) No more psychiatric labels: why formal psychiatric diagnostic systems should be abolished. *International Journal of Clinical and Health Psychology*, 14(3): 208–215.

Trimble MR & George MS (2010) *Biological Psychiatry*, 3rd edition. Chichester: Wiley-Blackwell.

Trivedi P (2010) A recovery approach in mental health services: transformation, tokenism or tyranny? In Basset T & Stickley T (eds) *Voices of Experience: Narratives of Mental Health Survivors*. Chichester: John Wiley & Sons, pp. 152–163.

Unzicker R (1989) On my own: a personal journey through madness and re-emergence. *Psychosocial Rehabilitation Journal*, 13(1): 71–77.

Van Hal G (2015) The true cost of the economic crisis on psychological well-being: a review. *Psychology Research and Behavior Management*, 8: 17–15.

van Os J (2016) 'Schizophrenia' does not exist. *British Medical Journal*, 352: i375.

Varese P, Smeets F, Drukker M ... Bentall RP (2012) Childhood adversities increase the risk of psychosis: a meta-analysis of patient-control, prospective- and cross-sectional cohort studies. *Schizophrenia Bulletin*, 38(4): 661–671.

Vaughan B, Goldstein MH, Alikakos M ... Serby MJ (2014) Frequency of reporting of adverse events in randomized controlled trials of psychotherapy vs. psychopharmacotherapy. *Comprehensive Psychiatry*, 55(4): 849–855.

Venkatasubramanian G & Keshavan MS (2016) Biomarkers in psychiatry – a critique. *Annals of Neurosciences*, 23(1): 3–5.

Walker C, Johnson K & Cunningham L (eds) (2012) *Community Psychology and the Socio-Economics of Mental Distress: International Perspectives*. Basingstoke: Palgrave Macmillan.

Wallcraft J (2015) Service-user-led research on psychosis: marginalisation and the struggle for progression. In Coles S, Keenan S & Diamond B (eds) *Madness Contested: Power and Practice*. Monmouth: PCCS Books, pp. 197–212.

Wallcraft J, Read J & Sweeney A (2003) *On Our Own Terms: Users and Survivors of Mental Health Services Working Together for Support and Change*. London: The Sainsbury Centre for Mental Health.

Wampold BE (2015) How important are the common factors in psychotherapy? An update. *World Psychiatry*, 14(3): 270–277.

Wampold BE & Imel ZE (2015) *The Great Psychotherapy Debate: The Evidence for What Makes Psychotherapy Work*, 2nd edition. New York, NY: Routledge.

Watson S, Thorburn K, Everett M & Fisher KR (2014) Care without coercion – mental health rights, personal recovery and trauma-informed care. *Australian Journal of Social Issues*, 49(4): 529–549.

Watters E (2011) *Crazy Like Us: The Globalization of the Western Mind*. London: Constable & Robinson.

Westmacott R & Hunsley J (2007) Weighing the evidence for psychotherapy equivalence: implications for research and practice. *The Behavior Analyst Today*, 8(2): 210–225.

Whitaker R (2015) *Anatomy of an Epidemic: Magic Bullets, Psychiatric Drugs, and the Astonishing Rise of Mental Illness in America*. New York, NY: Broadway Books.

Whitaker R & Cosgrove L (2015) *Psychiatry Under the Influence*. New York, NY: Palgrave Macmillan.

WHO (World Health Organization and the Calouste Gulbenkian Foundation) (2014) *Social Determinants of Mental Health*. Geneva: World Health Organization.

Whooley O (2010) Diagnostic ambivalence: psychiatric workarounds and the Diagnostic and Statistical Manual of Mental Disorders. *Sociology of Health & Illness*, 32(3): 452–469.

Wilkinson R & Pickett K (2010) *The Spirit Level: Why Equality is Better for Everyone.* London: Penguin.

Williams S (2016) *Recovering from Psychosis: Empirical Evidence and Lived Experience.* Abingdon: Routledge.

Woolliams M, Williams K, Butcher D & Pye J (2011) *Be More Critical! A Practical Guide for Health and Social Care Students,* 2nd edition. Oxford: Oxford Brookes University.

Wunderink L, Nieboer RM, Wiersma D ... Nienhuis FJ (2013) Recovery in remitted first-episode psychosis at 7 years of follow-up of an early dose reduction/discontinuation or maintenance treatment strategy: long-term follow-up of a 2-year randomized clinical trial. *JAMA Psychiatry,* 70(9): 913–920.

Zanarini MC & Wedig MM (2014) Childhood adversity and the development of borderline personality disorder. In Sharp C & Tackett JL (eds) *Handbook of Borderline Personality Disorder in Children and Adolescents.* New York, NY: Springer, pp. 265–276.

Zubin J, Oppenheimer G & Neugebauer R (1985) Degeneration theory and the stigma of schizophrenia. *Biological Psychiatry,* 20(11): 1145–1148.

Zubin J & Spring B (1977) Vulnerability: a new view of schizophrenia. *Journal of Abnormal Psychology,* 86(2): 103–126.

INDEX

Page numbers in **bold** indicate tables; page numbers in *italics* indicate illustrations.